Joan K. Parry, DSW

Social Work Theory and Practice with the Terminally Ill
Second Edition

Pre-publication
REVIEW . . .

"**T**his timely book offers the reader a sensitive and practical approach to working with people with terminal illness and their family members. It specifically focuses on the role of social workers, nurses, and other health care professionals and provides relevant case examples, an extensive bibliography, and definitions of terms used most often in work with the terminally ill. The reader will find much useful information about hospice care.

The most important chapters for me were Chapters 3 and 4 dealing with the interdisciplinary team and ways to work with the dying patient and his or her family. On the topic of team work the author recommends that although there may be a blurring of roles, the most important thing to recognize is that each member of the team has his or her sphere of talent. After providing views on both sides of the issue, the author raises a question for research: should the dying person be a member of the interdisciplinary team?

The challenge for the health care team is to help the patient and family face the inevitability of death and to help them prepare to 'let go' in a timely manner. Whether one wishes to focus on theory or practice, I recommend this excellent, caring book to anyone who wants to meet the challenges of working with the terminally ill and their survivors."

Jeanne A. Gill, PhD, LCSW
Adjunct Faculty,
San Diego State University,
School of Social Work;
Vice President, AASWG,
Southern California Chapter

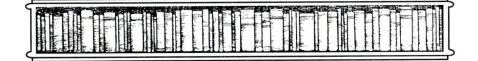

Social Work Theory and Practice with the Terminally Ill
Second Edition

Social Work Theory and Practice with the Terminally Ill
Second Edition

Joan K. Parry, DSW

The Haworth Social Work Practice Press
An Imprint of The Haworth Press, Inc.
New York • London • Oxford

Published by

The Haworth Social Work Practice Press, an imprint of The Haworth Press, Inc., 10 Alice Street, Binghamton, NY 13904-1580

Client identities and circumstances have been changed to protect confidentiality.

Cover design by Marylouise E. Doyle.

Library of Congress Cataloging-in-Publication Data

Parry, Joan K.
    Social work theory and practice with the terminally ill / Joan K. Parry.—2nd ed.
       p.   cm.
    Includes bibliographical references and index.
    ISBN 0-7890-1082-8 (hard : alk. paper)—ISBN 0-7890-1083-6 (soft : alk. paper)
    1. Social work with the terminally ill. 2. Social work with the terminally ill—United States.
I. Title.

HV3000 .P38 2000
362.1'75—dc21

00-038318

CONTENTS

ABOUT THE AUTHOR

Joan K. Parry, ACSW, LCSW, DSW, has 30 years of experience as a social work practitioner and teacher. She is Professor Emeritus from the San Jose State University School of Social Work. Dr. Parry served on the five-member National Task Force of the National Association of Social Workers to write continuing education standards for 100,000 professional social workers. She has held numerous other positions with NASW in both the New York and California state chapters and is also a member of the Council on Social Work Education. Dr. Parry is the author of several articles, chapters, and books, including the first edition of *Social Work Practice with the Terminally Ill* (1989) and *A Cross-Cultural Look at Death, Dying, and Religion* (1995).

Dr. Parry has worked as a psychiatric social worker at a mental health clinic, as a Family Service Supervisor in an all-black community, and as Director of Social Work at the Community Hospital in Glen Cove, New York. She taught at the Hunter College School of Social Work from 1980 to 1984, and the San Jose State University College of Social Work from 1985 to 1993. She then retired from teaching and remains in the San Diego area as an LCSW Consultant.

Preface

This revised edition points out the problems related to death and dying that have been most disturbing to the public. Drive-by shootings, random murders, and violence toward women and children are problems that are all too common today. A loved one dying young, or in a violent way at any age, is the most distressing experience for a family.

If we think about a time when death was considered a natural part of the life cycle, it often seems as if it were hundreds of years ago. However, it was less than eighty-five years ago: people died at home, with supportive family members present. There was community mourning to assist the survivors. Crying was acceptable and rituals helped surviving family members and friends to accept the loss of their loved one.

When a family loses a young parent or a child at any age, it is one of the most devastating experiences imaginable. It can take a long time to move beyond the pain and sadness created by the abrupt loss. This is compounded when the loss is due to a random act, such as being shot in crossfire between police and criminals; hit by a drunk driver; or gunned down in a school shooting because of your race, religion, or sexual orientation.

Hate crimes, school shootings, car accidents, drowning deaths, guns, and knives are all part of the current everyday lexicon in this country. Therefore, social workers in all settings will encounter family members who have experienced these horrendous losses, as well as those who have lost a loved one to a terminal illness. Sudden death can cause deep psychological and somatic pain. Terminal illness, although not desirable, gives most family members and loved ones some time to begin to process feelings of loss.

As previously stated, social workers can encounter individuals who have experienced the sudden death of a family member in almost any setting, including a child welfare agency, a family agency, an addiction service, almost anywhere. If the individual or family who seeks help for a problem has experienced a loss, the social worker needs to know. The loss is often the real problem rather than the presenting problem. It is not quite accepted in our culture to seek help for the death of a family member, although groups for widows and widowers, groups for family members of homicide victims, and all hospices provide bereavement services on an individual basis and in groups.

This revised book attempts to provide techniques and ideas to assist social work practitioners, nurse practitioners, and other helping persons who encounter dying persons or survivors of a loved one's death, sudden or otherwise. These techniques and ideas are applicable whether the dying person and/or survivors have their experience in an acute care hospital, a nursing home, a hospice, their own homes, the street, a car, or a school or business. Dying, especially sudden random death, is a stressful event in our society, and the survivors will benefit from caring services delivered in a timely manner.

Many more services and programs are available today than ten to fifteen years ago, particularly group services. However, professional social workers still need to direct survivors to these group programs. As social workers and other helping professionals understand the needs of family members who survive a loved one's terminal illness or sudden death, they will be better able to help persons who have experienced a powerful loss.

Joan K. Parry

Chapter 1

Current Situation

A social worker in a hospital setting was told that the accounts manager's secretary had been admitted with a diagnosis of cancer. The worker was anxious to see this patient, since they had had lunch together on occasion. The worker found the patient's room and opened the door. A woman with a gray pallor, sunken cheeks, and pinched lips was in the hospital bed, head propped up on two pillows. Her bony hands were crossed over her stomach, and her eyes were closed. The social worker stood at the door but could not go in.

ATTITUDES TOWARD DEATH

Although social workers in hospital settings have served dying patients and their families* throughout the years, the experience may create distress for these workers. Social workers' values and attitudes reflect societal norms and customs. Death is viewed by society as a feared intruder. The fact of death is avoided; youth, happiness, and health are expressed as eternal verities in American society. To die is to fail; to stop producing is to be untrue to the American ideal. American culture stresses the future, activity, and mastery of the environment; death stands in opposition to this spectrum of values.

Although social work has always been considered one of the helping professions, the workers themselves often avoid dealing

---

*Throughout this book, the general term family is used to include any significant person(s) in the dying individual's life.

1

with death. According to Ginzburg (1977), death does not fit the model for treating social problems in which such issues as poverty, disease, crime, loneliness, and interpersonal conflicts have the potential to respond to social work strategies of change. Although it can be handled intelligently and humanely, death is final, nonpreventable, universal, and irreversible. As a result, it requires a strategy of acceptance and adjustment.

We assume social roles as we grow from children to adults and thereby also take on a complex cluster of attitudes, beliefs, behaviors, and values. Thus, we are not only deeply socialized into the ways and norms of our culture but also represent and express these attitudes and values in every form of our conduct. The nurses' cluster of attitudes, beliefs, values, and behaviors tell them that it is wrong to grieve in public, that it is correct to "hold in" their feelings. The family members' cluster of attitudes, beliefs, values, and conduct may tell them that the only response to sudden loss is keening. Zaner (1985, p. 228) comments that to live in a social world is to live an ordered and meaningful life within the embrace of an overarching "social nomos" (order, rule, law). However, the orders, rules, and laws of behavior and conduct are shaped and molded by the culture in which we are reared. The crisis of sudden death is an experience that is processed with various mechanisms and elicits various responses. It is important to understand that family life issues are much more complex today, and in a sudden-death or terminal-illness situation, the social worker must attend to these complexities.

Bereavement groups are very helpful to persons who feel at sea after a loss and who are at higher risk for morbidity and mortality. Men and women struggle with changes such as being single after being part of a couple, and loneliness manifests itself when an individual does minor, routine activities alone that were previously done together.

However, the possibility of personal growth always exists. Since most of those bereaved due to loss of a spouse are women, the new responsibilities and roles force them to become involved in new behaviors. It can involve new jobs, changing the home inside and out, or moving to a new location. The process of personal growth and change for men and women also influences the decision about how to deal with the personal effects of the deceased. The ability to dispose of personal effects can suggest acceptance of the loss or perhaps the dismissal of a spouse for whom one felt a good deal of ambivalence. The bereavement group struggles with the tension between the process of change and a sense of devotion to the deceased spouse.

In general, a group for widows and widowers helps members to share their experiences with others. Thus, group meetings help individuals cope with the social isolation that is often pervasive for bereaved spouses, but as stated earlier, they also assist members in reaching an understanding of the changes facing them and to experience growth as well as acute loss. Yolom and Vinogrador (1988) found that bereavement groups, rather than dwelling on loss, pain, or emotional catharsis, concentrate on growth, self-knowledge, and existential responsibility.

Death is final and irreversible, but dying is a process, and much change and growth can occur during that process for the patient, the family, and the social worker. Sudden death, however, does not allow time for a process, and the worker's interventions must be concentrated on the survivors. Work with survivors is also a process, whether they have suffered loss from lingering or sudden death. Reality is that all our lives are fragile. Someday we will die, and before we die, we are likely to face the death of others whom we love (DiGiulio and Krantz, 1995, p. 24).

EFFECTS OF INSTITUTIONALIZATION

In addition to the discomfort social workers may feel in working with dying patients, the nature of institutional settings often contributes to the problems workers may encounter.

Institutionalization itself is often conceptualized by researchers as a dehumanizing experience. Dying in an institution can exacerbate physical and psychological problems of chronic pain, fear, dependency, and loss of self-esteem. Rabin and Rabin (1985) said hospitals are apt to deteriorate into dehumanized machines. The first thing that patients experience when they enter the hospital is a loss of personal identity. A woman could be referred to as "that case of uterine cancer in the bed near the door," not as Mary Jones. The disease is treated, but Mary Jones is lying awake at night worrying about her husband and her children. Feifel (1977, p. 7) noted that medical advances have lengthened the average time that elapses between the onset of a fatal illness and death. Medical practice has also altered the focus of dying. We no longer die in the privacy and security of our homes, but in a hospital or nursing home, "where our lot is the death of a sickness rather than a person" (Feifel, 1977, p. 7). Although statistics pertaining to deaths in institutions as opposed to deaths at home are scarce, it is known that from 1949 to 1958 a 10 percent increase occurred nationwide in deaths in institutions, including general hospitals and nursing homes. New York City statistics reveal a 7 percent decrease in deaths at home from 1955 to 1967. This trend continued for cancer, in which 30 percent of such deaths occurred at home in 1959; by 1979, only 15 percent of cancer deaths were at home (Mor and Hiris, 1983). There have been ongoing inquiries examining the site of death and the way people die, including hospice (Parliament of Victoria, 1987). Mor (1987) pointed out in a discussion of hospice that the focus on home care, dehospitalization, and a shift in caretaking responsibility from the institution to the family all helped sell the hospice concept to a parsimonious Congress. There is evidence that deaths in institutions have been rapidly replacing deaths at home in the thirty years after World War II (Ryder and Ross, 1977). These statistics suggest that dying in one's home is harder to achieve than dying in an institution. It must be kept in mind, however, that most children and adults in today's world are not often exposed to death and are more comfortable taking their sick relatives to the hospital to die.

It is not surprising that adults have difficulty coping with death (Friel, 1985); even families who have expressed the desire to have their loved one die at home often find the final days too much to bear and take their dying family member to the hospital. Conversely, it is also sometimes the case, particularly in today's hospital climate, that families are urged to take patients home even though the family may not feel ready to do so.

The following case example illustrates some of these problems and ways in which the social worker can intervene:

Mrs. D. cried a little when she saw the social worker in the hospital the first working day of the new year. She thought that when her husband fell down on New Year's Eve it was from drinking too much alcohol, but after a weekend in bed and a trip to the neurologist, Mr. D. was hospitalized. His speech had become blurred, and three days after he was admitted, brain surgery was performed. Two tumors were found; one had burst, and another was inoperable. He was given radiation treatments, and the oncologist told Mrs. D. that he had twelve to eighteen months to live. Mr. D. was unavailable to the social worker because he had reacted with excessive hostility, a by-product of the brain tumor. Mrs. D. was too frantic to use the social worker effectively, even though the social worker was able to take in her sadness and anger. Yet, initially, Mrs. D. was able to use concrete help to take Mr. D. home.

Mr. D. returned home in early March. A nurse was hired for the daytime. Mrs. D. worked. Their two sons, who were eleven and thirteen years old, attended school. Mr. D.'s mother was also present. At night, she and Mrs. D. took care of Mr. D. She told the social worker he often insisted on getting up and going to the bathroom, and then he could never make it back. Mrs. D. would have to go outside and find two strong men to get him back in bed. She said he continued to react to his illness with anger and physical violence. Mrs. D. commented, "He is thirty-nine years old, weighs 240 pounds, and is a big strong man who is used to carrying everyone on his back." Mr. D. died in early May.

This case illustrates a sudden onset of terminal illness that created chaos for the patient and the family members. In the present hospital climate, with diagnosis-related groups (DRGs) dictating lengths of hospital stay, many patients such as Mr. D. are being sent home. Patients with considerable dementia, such as Mr. D. had, or PWAs (persons with AIDS), are not in need of acute hospital care, but institutionalization would probably be more helpful to the family. Conversely, if the dying person is fully cognizant of the situation, institutionalization can create added emotional stress. The social worker helped with ventilation of feelings and home care arrangements and made it clear to Mrs. D. that she was always available. This allowed Mrs. D. to return for follow-up help many months after Mr. D. died. The social worker was able to ameliorate to some degree the dissonance of hospitalization for Mrs. D.

INSTITUTIONAL CHARACTERISTICS

The acute care hospital is characterized by a hierarchical structure, with the physician at the apex of a system of medical care bound by routines and schedules. This is emphasized by Hamric (1977), who comments that the hospital mission is to keep things running smoothly. Routine becomes a barrier to humanistic care. The rigid hierarchical structure with the physician at the top of the team tends to make other members, such as nurses and social workers, feel as if death is a team failure (Hamric, 1977). The skilled nursing facility is also an organizational arrangement in which a hierarchical structure is present, but the nurse or the administrator is at the top. Although routines are less rigid, boredom and inertia are often connected to a long-term care facility. The hospice provides a type of care for the terminally ill in a nonbureaucratic place where routines are minimal, but individuals such as Mr. D. rarely become hospice patients.

Dissonance of Institutional Care vis-à-vis the Patient

The dissonance of institutional care vis-à-vis the dying patient and the family was not fully recognized in the United States until the book *On Death and Dying* by Elisabeth Kübler-Ross was published in 1969. Before the publication of the Kübler-Ross book, not discussing a person's prognosis or illness with him or her may have been motivated by a desire to spare the sick person. This has changed to keeping quiet about dying to spare society. Death was seen as shameful and forbidding (Rabin and Rabin, 1985). Dying persons were put in hospitals or nursing homes to keep them out of sight. Institutionalization was often equated with avoidance of the subject of dying and the discomforts associated with it. The Kübler-Ross book served as a catalyst for the submerged concerns of the public and many health care workers. As she points out, we were in the middle of the Vietnam War, and physicians were seeing more dying patients with emotional problems, whose needs could best be met by social workers and chaplains. The book arrived on fertile ground and created a rush of interest in the themes of listening and caring for dying patients.

In the institutional setting, a dying patient may feel isolated, fearful, and abandoned. The family may withdraw, deny the reality of the illness, or indulge in behavior to prevent talking about the dying experience either among themselves or with the patient. This was, in effect, the way Mrs. D. responded to the sudden and overwhelming experience of her husband's critical illness.

There is a caveat, however, and that is with high-profile persons in hospitals who have been shot in a school, or people hit by a drunk driver who is high profile, or people who are attacked or mutilated. These high-profile persons are burdened with too much attention. Today, many people live in gated communities or have extra locks on their doors and perimeter security systems around their homes. According to Flannery (1997), violence in America has become a national public health problem of epidemic proportion. The question raised here is how health workers react to much of this wanton violence, the results of which often appear in hospital emergency rooms. The initial reaction to such violence is professionalism and care for the persons who need it, followed by fear. Health workers know that the same random violence could happen to them or their loved ones, and that is a fear-provoking thought.

Effect of Behaviors of Health Care Workers

The latent fears that most of us share concerning death are heightened by the illness and expected death of others. When health care workers, including social workers, assume postures of denial, oversolicitousness, and hyperobjectivity, it may reflect an inner desire to be dissociated from the reality of death. Such behaviors by social workers and other health care staff are stark reminders to the patient of his or her apartness from others. When faced with such rejecting responses, the patient is forced to develop defenses such as total denial or secondary gain, which further exacerbate the person's lack of emotional and physical well-being (Henderson, 1972). Mr. D.'s anger and hostility can be cited as one example of these defenses.

If the health care staff is not prepared for the many complexities and demands of the dying patient, staff members may resist responding to the nonphysical needs of the patient. They deny their own discomfort with death by avoiding the patient and expressing excessive concern with maintaining routines.

The result of avoidance behaviors by health care staff is to close channels of communication among patient, family, and social worker; to reduce flexibility of caring functions; to separate family from the patient; to lose sight of symptom control; and to reduce the ability of social workers to intervene in meaningful ways. Instead, energy is displaced onto medical debates about death. When does it occur? What is brain death, heart stoppage, etc.? Should death be avoided at all costs? Should it be allowed to occur more rapidly? Who should make the decisions about whether to prolong or shorten life? These discussions are a kind of death denial and have little relevance outside of the institutional setting.

It would appear that in the case of Mr. D.'s terminal illness, medical personnel did not give Mrs. D. the time or consideration she needed to deal with a frightening and overwhelming situation. The physician in charge was not able to handle the family members' situation in a personal, caring way.

The social worker is often aware that the physicians' sense of omnipotence is a key component in the way they react to terminally ill patients and their families. This is particularly apparent with cancer patients, for, in many of these cases, physicians are unable to cure and, therefore, feel they have lost their powers (Schnaper, Kellner, and Koeppel, 1985, p. 87). The diagnosis may create physician hostility toward the patient and/or family because of the inexorable fact of death, which threatens the physician's feelings of omnipotence.

Some of these attitudes and feelings of physicians and other health professionals are developed during their professional schooling. It is worthwhile to summarize Sinacore's (1981) study on the subject of attitudes of a spectrum of health professionals who work with dying patients. He hypothesizes that the unspoken part of the health curriculum focuses on the technical aspects of death, and these covert influences arise from the use of the medical model, the language of the health professional, and the expectation of the medicalized patient. The human condition is inadvertently taken out of the realm of social meaning. The impending death is viewed as a chronic challenge to life, and, thus, the patient is met with increased technological management. The focus of care for that terminally ill patient is scientific, not humanistic.

Institutional Constraints

The issue of institutional constraints must be considered. Constraints are the need to move people out of the hospital because of reimbursement requirements and the excessive paperwork required to support actions taken by health care workers, including social workers. Administrators are mostly concerned about reimbursement and malpractice. Lohmann (1979) has commented that contemporary social institutions provide inadequate support for staff working with dying patients and families. He conducted a survey of a number of social workers in acute care hospitals who attempted to provide counseling services to the terminally ill. Those interviewed reported that they were frequently frustrated in their efforts by a lack of official recognition and sanction.

Considerable change has occurred in the last ten years, particularly with the advent of Medicare coverage for hospice service. Some institutions undoubtedly still constrain those serving terminally ill patients, but as hospitals move more and more into the home care business, more attention will be paid to the dying patient. An ongoing concern is the relationship of hospice care to the medical care system (McDonnell, 1986). Two extremes are suggested, one of which is a totally separate system for the care of the terminally ill, apart from and unrelated to the rest of health care. The other extreme is for hospice care to be completely absorbed into the general medical care system. Neither of these extremes is acceptable, but, rather, it is hoped that a middle ground will be established in which the management of dying patients will, in some respects, be a specialty, but one that fits comfortably into the framework of the traditional medical care system (McDonnell, 1986, p. 203).

In complex health care organizations a dilemma may arise, since the organization is oriented to serving the collective interests of all its patients, which demands that the interests of some clients must be sacrificed. As a result, professional social workers who want to develop a model of care for dying patients and families (described later) may be in conflict with the interest of the organization. Hospitals and skilled nursing facilities are complex organizations, and the hospice is an evolving complex organization. The nature of the institutional structures, procedures, and administrative interests in the three types of health care organizations impacts on how social workers approach their work with terminally ill patients and their families. Strauss, Glaser, and Quint (1964, pp. 73-74) concur and comment that "hospital policies profoundly influence how personnel respond to terminal patients." They add that the emphasis in hospitals and other institutional settings is on physical needs, even though the more pressing need is for psychological services (p. 74).

Therefore, in the hospital and skilled nursing facility, where most people die, the dying are given low priority on resources. The status of dying patients in these institutional settings is lowered and can reduce care, which may either hasten death or prolong it unnecessarily. If care plans of the institution are directed away from terminally ill patients, this will affect ways in which the social workers perceive the institutional care provided and their own attitudes and feelings about their jobs and clients. Germain (1980, p. 80) writes that the health care organization may exert constraints on the social worker's ability to respond flexibly and effectively to patient and family needs, or it may offer opportunities to provide excellent service, or, more likely, it will be a mixture of constraint and opportunities.

Likert (1967, p. 47) discusses effective organizations that use supportive relationships, group decision making, group methods of supervision, and high expectations. The organization must ensure a maximum opportunity for each member to view his or her experience as supportive, which builds and maintains a sense of personal worth and importance.

MODEL OF CARE FOR THE TERMINALLY ILL

A perceived ideal model for the institutional care of the terminally ill includes five elements: (1) open communication, (2) flexible facilities, (3) patient/family as a unit of care, (4) symptom control, and (5) interdisciplinary team (Parry, 1983). The model can work in various institutional settings, such as hospitals, skilled nursing facilities, and hospices. The five elements are defined in the following sections.

Open Communication

Open communication facilitates trust among the patient, family, and health care team. The issue is not whether "to tell" or "not to tell" but, rather, sharing information. Open communication allows health staff to be available to listen if and when the patient or family feels like talking about the dying experience. Honest and sensitive communication from the social worker and other health professionals about the gravity of a patient's condition tends to attenuate feelings of guilt and inadequacy, not only in the patient but in professional personnel and family as well.

Flexible Facilities

With flexible facilities, it is assumed that patients need to be involved in making decisions about their care. If patients feel free to ask questions, and if they receive information about care as desired, they take an active part in decisions about their physical surroundings so that their needs or wishes for a homelike atmosphere are fulfilled. Such an atmosphere includes their own furniture (in their living room or hospital room), pets, and visitors, as desired. Flexibility to create a homelike and supportive environment reduces feelings of helplessness and dependency.

Patient/Family As a Unit of Care

Social work has always viewed the family as a unit. Therefore, if one member becomes sick, all other members of the family are affected. Terminal illness upsets the equilibrium of the family group. As a result, time spent listening empathically to a family member who has aches and pains is perceived as productive for family and patient. As the dying person becomes more disabled, the family must provide both physical and emotional support. Scholars have said that families need to be involved in caregiving because as a terminal disease progresses, family members become increasingly important contributors to the quality of life for the dying person. Families can become part of the care team with terminal patients (Goldstein, 1973; Gonda and Ruark, 1984). Not only do family members need care, but they also need to be involved in caregiving, either at home or in the institutional setting.

Symptom Control

Symptoms can become the overriding concern of the terminally ill patient and can run the gamut from severe, chronic physical pain to overconcern about the ability to fill out insurance forms. There can be social, emotional, spiritual, physical, interpersonal, and financial distress in the dying experience. Each symptom should be treated as a separate entity and given more than routine attention. If symptoms are perceived to be controlled and help is given in the areas needed, it is assumed, by the individual patient, the family members, and the health team, that there will be time to work through the meaning of life and dying. Krant (1972, p. 101) states that if the patient is helped to "die well," the meaning of terminal illness changes for the patient, the family, and the staff.

Interdisciplinary Team

The ideal health team is a joint effort in which individual members bring their special talents, training, skills, and expertise to the caring situation. This kind of team has regular communications, the ability to use one another for mutual support, and a strong sense of egalitarianism among team members. Dying patients and their families have multifaceted problems with physical, psychological, legal, social, spiritual, economic, and interpersonal ramifications. Therefore, the situation requires the collaboration of many disciplines working as an integrated clinical team. The team should meet frequently to discuss patient care planning and for mutual staff support. Interdependence and interrelatedness are developed through formal meetings and shared crises.

Caplan (1974, p. 132) comments that social workers, by virtue of their training in self-awareness, are best able to assist other team members to admit and accept emotional disequilibrium, not only in patients and families but also among the staff members themselves. Caplan states further, "It is a source of great relief to an individual team member to know that the group will help him to avoid transferring onto his relationship with his client his own disequilibrium of the moment."

THE HOSPICE MOVEMENT

Hospice is an organizational arrangement that could meet Likert's test for effectiveness. Hospice is not a new idea. In fact, the modern hospice can be traced to a co-worker of Florence Nightingale, Sister Mary Aiken, head of the Irish Sisters of Charity, who opened a hospice in Dublin in the late nineteenth century (Seplowin and Seravilli, 1983). St. Joseph's Hospice was established by the English Sisters of Charity in London in 1906 (Stoddard, 1978). It was at St. Joseph's during the 1950s and 1960s that Dr. Cicely Saunders conducted her work in pain control and made plans for St. Christopher's Hospice, which opened in 1967. Dr. Saunders developed the modern concept of hospice in England in the 1960s. In 1948, she was a medical social worker when she became concerned about the kinds of care provided to dying patients. She returned to school and studied to become a physician so she could gain knowledge about pain and help dying patients in more concrete ways. Saunders worked many years to gain support, both moral and financial, to build St. Christopher's Hospice in London.

The hospice concept took root in the United States in the early 1970s. Zelda Foster, an American social worker, was a member of the International Work Group on Death and Dying, which met in 1974, 1976, and 1978 and helped to develop standards for hospice care (Foster, 1979).

Hospice care moved to North America in January 1975 with the opening of the Palliative Care Unit at the Royal Victoria Hospital in Montreal. At the same time, Hospice Incorporated of Connecticut was beginning operations in the New Haven area. In 1978, the Comptroller General of the United States reported that fifty-nine hospices were operating in the United States. A year later, Cohen (1979) listed more than 200 hospices in different stages of development in this country. When the new Medicare regulations for hospice care were enacted in 1983, *The New York Times* (1983) reported an estimated 1,200 hospices. In 1985 it was estimated that 1,694 hospices were operational (Mor, 1987). There were over 2,100 hospices in the United States in 1995 (Bernard and Schneider, 1996, p. 13).

Hospices are organized in many different forms: home care only, hospital-based with dedicated beds or wing, scattered hospital beds with a rotating hospice team, skilled nursing facility with dedicated beds, or freestanding hospice unit. All hospices, whether in a hospital, nursing home, or freestanding, have home care components. The team is basically composed of a physician, nurse, social worker, and clergy member. Other members can include a psychiatrist, psychologist, nutritionist, pharmacist, health aide, administrator, radiation therapist, occupational therapist, recreation therapist, and family members; there is always a cadre of dedicated volunteers.

Hospice is one attempt to respond with humanistic care to the needs of the terminally ill. Although not all terminally ill patients can be served by hospice, it is a concept that can use support by the health community.

The following principles are embedded in the standards for accreditation for hospices (Mor, 1987):

- The patient and family are the unit of care.
- Interdisciplinary team services available to the patient and family must include at least physician, nursing, psychological/social work, spiritual, volunteer, and bereavement services.
- Intervention focuses on the management of physical and psychological symptoms.
- Hospice service must be available twenty-four hours a day, seven days a week.
- Inpatient services must be available as well as home care, and continuity of care across both settings must be assured.

These standards have evolved over a fifteen-year period. The hospice movement has been part of a general death awareness, emphasis on emotional needs, and reaction against technological medicine and the institutionalization of death. This, combined with a focus on consumer rights that encouraged the right of the individual to participate in decision making and negative reactions to institutionalization, paved the way for an enthusiastic reception of the hospice movement in the United States.

Social workers are, or should be, core members of the hospice team. Social workers have the opportunity to be an integral part of the interdisciplinary team in a hospice setting. In hospitals, they may participate in teams at various times, but not in an ongoing way and rarely as core members. The bereavement services in hospice are frequently coordinated by social workers; community education and staff in-service are other hospice tasks that can be done by social workers. Social workers are represented as professional staff in 58 to 63 percent of hospice programs (Mor, 1987). The concept envisions staff as using supportive relationships, group decision making, group methods of supervision, and maintaining high expectations about the service to the patient/family. Social workers who are employed in hospices are assumed to be familiar with, and comfortable with, the terminally ill patient and the patient's family.

Mrs. D. could have made good use of a hospice volunteer in the home when Mr. D. was discharged, and later, to help her get her life together.

Mrs. D. shared with the social worker that she had attended a widow's group for ten weeks, and it helped her to understand her family's feelings—particularly those of her youngest son, who had never cried and was difficult to handle and angry all the time. Her oldest son had cried when his father became very sick and sobbed when he died. Mrs. D. said that she did not have time to cry, and Mr. D.'s mother cried all the time. She said that her youngest son was like a little boy, and her oldest son had taken over his father's place. Perhaps a hospice volunteer could have been helpful to these two boys in working through the loss of their father.

Although most hospice programs are under medical direction, there is an effort toward teamwork and a push for active participation by the patient and family. Symptom control is more important than exotic medical intervention. The stated hospice principles are closely allied with social work values and norms, such as respect for individuality, self-determination, integrity of person and family, and the right to humanistic caring.

The Hospice Since Medicare

Congress provided Medicare benefits for hospice patients beginning in 1984. The program provided a standard of hospice care for anyone eligible for Social Security Medicare. The insurance industry used a similar model of care to provide services to those under sixty-five. The standards allow people who wish to die at home to do so. Hospice care uses the services of a team that is typically made up of the dying individual, family members, caregivers, referring primary care physician, nurses, home health aides, physical therapists, occupational therapists, chaplains, volunteers, and social workers (Bernard and Schneider, 1996, p. 19).

The Medicare benefit sets up a systematic way to provide care, stating who shall give care, at what time, and in what way. Services can occur at home, in a hospital, in a skilled nursing facility, in a freestanding hospice, and even on city streets, if care involves the homeless. The level of need dictates the care, which may require only a volunteer to give respite to family members, a nurse for pain management, or a social worker for emotional needs. Other patients and families need the whole team.

Medicare also provides the patient with medical equipment such as oxygen, a hospital bed, a wheelchair, etc. Medications to provide pain relief and comfort are supplied. Basically, Medicare attempts to provide the services needed to alleviate physical, emotional, and spiritual distress.

SOCIAL WORKERS AND TERMINAL ILLNESS

Social workers have interacted with dying persons from the beginning of social work practice in hospitals. This type of social work began at Massachusetts General Hospital in 1905. Cabot (1915, 1919) describes the social work service, including some discussion of dying patients, in two books. Later, Bartlett (1961) refers to the experience of working with dying patients as an inherent element of social work practice in medical settings. Social work with the terminally ill has never been described as an easy task.

Social workers have been involved in the development of a body of knowledge in thanatology, which is the study of death and its psychological and social implications. They have also participated in a movement for humanistic care in response to the impersonal technological resources of large medical institutions where control has shifted from patient and family to the institution.

SUMMARY

In our society, we often perceive death and dying as a sign of failure. In this setting, social workers often have trouble relating to the dying patient. Health care workers in the institutional setting may avoid or deny the fact of death when dealing with terminally ill patients. The model of care presented in this chapter can be used to effectively help dying patients and their families. The hospice concept can be used to provide humanistic care for dying patients. The social worker who has first faced his or her own fears and attitudes toward death can then enter the room of a dying person as an effective health care professional and a caring human being.

Chapter 2

Defining Terminal Illness

The moment of diagnosis, the treatment phase, the hospitalization, the increase of medical personnel in one's life—all are part of the definition of terminal illness. Kalish (1971, p. 1) comments that "dying is an adjective that describes a set of circumstances faced by a living individual." A person who is defined as being terminally ill is living, although living can present multiple problems. The patient can become frustrated by the persistence and exacerbation of his or her physical discomfort and by the pain that may accompany the disease or treatment process.

A fifteen-year-old adolescent recently diagnosed with leukemia must cope with the sense of immortality and invincibility that were her prerogatives as a healthy young girl. She must also cope with enormous changes in her daily life, since she will be attending a clinic instead of going to school until she achieves remission after rigorous and painful treatment (Bender, 1987).

Sometimes in the field of thanatology, death and dying are lumped together as if they were one entity. Each terminally ill person is an individual who experiences his or her illness in a unique way. The brain tumor for Mr. D. is very different from Hodgkin's disease in another person. The terminally ill are not a homogeneous group. Each person brings to his or her illness a specific tumor or disease diagnosis of varying type and extent, individual manifestations of the disease, individual reactions to the disease, family, friends, and the awareness of impending death. These are dynamic pieces of the whole picture that create constant change in the patient's medical and emotional status.

COPING PATTERNS OF THE TERMINALLY ILL

Initial Reaction

It would seem that a part of the definition of terminal illness would include the individual's initial reaction to the news of the life-threatening condition. Shock, numbness, outright denial, anger, fear, and sadness are common specific reactions to being informed that one has a life-threatening illness (Gonda and Ruark, 1984).

Such news can make patients and family members stuporous, and clinicians who do not heed this shock to the involved parties will often find they are talking to themselves. Persons numbed by news of a terminal diagnosis can no longer process what is being said to them. The clinician should know it can be helpful to provide a reflection of their feelings to patients and families: "This must be overwhelming to you," or "Perhaps you need time to digest this news, and then you can ask the questions you want answered." Such supportive statements may or may not penetrate the numbness, but the statements and the feelings that accompany them will help to build a trusting relationship.

Denial and Anger

Denial is protective and is discussed in greater detail at the conclusion of this chapter. Suffice it to say that statements from patients and families which suggest that they do not believe the doctor, or that they believe the doctor made a mistake, are deflecting the information until they can regroup and begin to process the shocking medical information. This goes hand in hand with anger, which is the other side of denial. Anger at the bearer of bad tidings is understandable and to be expected; in fact, it may spill out onto all members of the health care team. However, anger may provide the necessary energy needed to cope with the disagreeable unfolding of the illness.

Fear

Fear comes when the numbness abates and denial stops working in service of the ego. Fear can immobilize a person, or it can marshal the strengths, if necessary, to fight the feared intruder. Gonda and Ruark (1984, p. 89) comment that an ability to connect to the appropriate primordial reaction, such as fear, may reflect psychological strength.

Sadness

Sadness at the initial news of one's illness is usually defined as depression. As the reality of the illness sets in, many losses occur, including a job, planned vacations, future events, loss of freedom caused by frequent hospitalizations or constant medical treatment, and financial worries. This depression is a reaction to the threat and the consequences of an illness. Depression also occurs later in the illness. This is the anticipatory grief related to the patient's preparation for separation from life. According to Friel (1985, p. 175), the patient is in the process of losing everything and everyone he or she loves, and it is only natural that such a threat should evoke sadness. It may help to dissipate the first type of depression. The second and final sadness should be accepted and expressed by both patients and families. This can be equated with Kübler-Ross's (1969) final stage of acceptance, as described in her seminal book *On Death and Dying*. A caveat is in order: not every dying patient experiences acceptance. The different reactions of dying persons are described as discrete phenomena for the purpose of understanding the varying feelings and experiences that can occur for each person.

MODELS OF THE DYING TRAJECTORY

Zimmerman (1981, p. 14) defines terminal illness as that situation in which antitumor therapy does not offer a reasonable possibility of cure. He is describing hospice patients, who are usually cancer patients. He also includes in his definition a life expectancy of less than six months. This is the definition used for including dying persons in a hospice program. It is a somewhat arbitrary time frame needed to determine whether an individual meets hospice eligibility criteria. Often the persons who come to hospice have only days or hours left to live.

Persons who are diagnosed with tumors, blood disease, kidney failure, and the like sometimes live for years before death occurs. In many of these situations, the individual is confronted with a life-threatening illness that presents great uncertainty. Life threatening means the disease is capable of ending life, but in what length of time is uncertain. This is what Pattison (1977, p. 44) refers to as "the crisis of knowledge of death." He sets up a paradigm of the "dying trajectory" in which the crisis of knowledge of death creates a peak anxiety and an acute crisis phase. This crisis is followed by a second phase, the chronic living-dying phase, which is the longest, lasting for days, weeks, months, or years. This phase is character-ized by periods of remission and exacerbation of the disease. Hope and despair are intermingled, and as the time between remission and exacerbation decreases, depression increases. A third phase, the terminal phase, is not precise but begins when the dying person starts to withdraw in response to body signals.

This withdrawal phenomenon has been noted by other writers and elaborated upon in other conceptual models relating to the timing of death. One such model is presented by Calkins (1971, p. 84), who suggests that most patients are admitted to a medical setting for the final stage of dying. In her formulation, this hospital admittance is initially perceived by the caretaker(s) as a medical emergency to keep the patient alive and then develops into the last stages of the patient's dying. For the family, social death occurs when the initial emergency has turned into a lingering dying experience: "Conse-quently, the patient has essentially died at the point when the family's interest changes from hoping he can be pulled through to questioning 'Why don't they let him die?'"

Social Death

The concept of social death is much broader than that of biologi-cal death. Some patients are elderly and have limited or no family. If they need long-term care due to debilitating illness, they are often socially dead to those persons who are the health caretakers. Staff members make fine distinctions among patients under their care: there are degrees of dementia; there are also degrees of likability. Staff can become attached if patients are not completely demented. Glaser and Strauss (1968) stated that both personnel and family are effectively protected against a sense of deep loss by their judgments that these patients' lives no longer have much value to themselves, to their families, or to the larger society. This lack of value of life is always related to elderly persons. One can hear, "He was so old," "She lived a long life," or "He's better off dead." Deaths are written off, and patients in long-term care facilities may feel socially dead even though they may be in relatively good health. Thus, it is double jeopardy to be terminally ill and to be elderly. Health personnel who perceive these patients as people without value then deprive them of their humanity, creating social death.

An understanding of social death allows the social worker to intervene to change the deadly impact of this phenomenon. Noting the change in relatives' attitudes toward the dying patient is important for the social worker involved with family and patient. The social worker knows this terminal phase can last hours, days, or weeks. Sometimes if the terminal phase is too brief, there may be recriminations on the part of the home caregivers: either they should have allowed the patient to die at home or the medical intervention was not good enough to help. When the dying experience is extended, or even brief recovery occurs, caregivers may become distressed because their expectations, in terms of the timing of the death, are not met.

The Nature of Death

Death is a state and dying is an event/process, but we can consider them as a unitary concept. There are several ways to symbolize death. The first and most fundamental is the perception of death as the end of life. The second could be what we call social death, or loss of vitality, and the potential for suicide. The third is that death can be equated with disaster, holocaust, ethnic cleansing, and genocide. The imagery of the second part of the twentieth century was filled with horrific death such as nuclear annihilation and famine (Rwanda, Yugoslavia, Cambodia) or death caused by individuals, as in school shootings, drunk driving, and so on. Due to media stress, the relationship between these types of sudden and unnatural death make death an ever-present reality in our lives.

But the individual dying in a hospital setting, whether from gunshot wound or cancer, exists in a cold, sterile environment in most hospitals. The "problem" of death seems to be one for technicians and experts rather than family members. Family members are not encouraged to gather and be able to say good-bye in their own ways. "It is our strong belief that it is time to reintroduce the love of family and the power of the home—even if, at times, only symbolically—into the heart of the process of dying" (Bernard and Schneider, 1996, p. 30).

The importance of these perceptions of death varies substantially, particularly relative to the issue of death as natural or unnatural. "But death, for the human imagination, never ceases to be a many-sided, seemingly contradictory yet ultimately unitary psychological form" (Lifton, 1979, p. 47).

CASE HISTORIES

Mr. F. died at age sixty-seven in a hospital less than twenty-four hours after being admitted. His blood condition had been diagnosed seven years earlier (the crisis of knowledge of death). After surgical correction of an eye dysfunction that identified the illness, he had five years relatively free of disease. However, more than two years before his death, he was hospitalized with a high fever and the possibility of impending death. At this point the social worker became involved with Mrs. F., who reacted to the sudden unexpected change in her husband's illness with overwhelming fear and anxiety. The social worker saw Mrs. F. on a weekly basis outside the hospital. Mr. F. stabilized and was discharged to home two weeks after hospitalization. However, he now needed bimonthly transfusions to maintain his life. Approximately two months after discharge, Mr. F. began to accompany Mrs. F. to the weekly sessions with the social worker.

Although Mr. and Mrs. F. lived with death as a certainty, they lacked a clear indication of time of death and mode of death. Yet the certainty of death was based on various clues, such as physical symptoms and medical tests (Glaser and Strauss, 1968). Mr. F.'s physical symptoms were shortness of breath and greatly reduced mobility. After discharge from the hospital, Mr. F. could not walk more than one-half block. Gradually, over eighteen months, his mobility was restricted to a few feet, then to a chair stair lift that was installed because he could not climb the stairs to his bedroom. His medical tests confirmed the diagnosis of myelofibrosis. Mr. F., an artist, had taught in the fine arts department at a college. Medical staff conjectured that his blood disease was the result of excessive exposure to open vats of benzene. The disease manifested itself with precipitous drops in blood hemoglobin and chronic oxygen insufficiency.

Mr. F. was in the chronic-dying phase of his illness for two years. It is during this phase of an illness that the social worker's intervention can be most meaningful. It must be stated that two years is an inordinately long period to have to help the patient and family members resolve problems and come to terms with the outcome. Social workers enable those with illnesses to discuss their feelings about dying, to talk about close family members and how they feel about them, and to strategize on how to discuss their feelings and physical discomforts with doctors. If time allows, workers can assist with family meetings to sort out communication problems. Social workers also help dying people work on their grief feelings and find better ways to cope with the activities of daily living. At times, providing concrete services, such as assisting with insurance forms, is very helpful as well.

Tasks of the Social Worker

Still, whether the time period involved is two years or two months, steps can be taken to enhance an individual's life during this chronic living-dying phase. If the dying person can learn to endure the losses, both physical and emotional, where grief is defined and accepted, then the dying person may tolerate loss of bodily functions and self-control, and control can be exercised where feasible. Dying persons can retain dignity and self-respect in the face of the terminating life cycle if they can place their lives in perspective within their own personal history, family, and tradition (Pattison, 1977).

This is the task the social worker assumed when she began working with Mr. and Mrs. F. Although some sessions were taken up with symptoms, reactions to transfusions, and medical appointments, there was a constant theme of life review, both as individuals and jointly. They had been married for forty years and had five adult children and several grandchildren.

In contrast to the case history of Mr. F., the following case history describes a woman whose death occurred much more quickly. Mrs. K. was a forty-five-year-old mother of nine children ranging in age from fourteen to twenty-eight years. Her husband had abandoned her four years earlier, and she was the main wage earner and caretaker of the four remaining minor children. She was hospitalized for relief from cranial pressure resulting from an earlier automobile accident. It was her third hospitalization for cranial relief. She made an unremarkable recovery after brain surgery and was ready to be discharged when several hard lumps were noticed on her neck. The neurosurgeon called another physician, who in turn had the patient undergo some medical tests. She was terrified of the tests and knew she had cancer before the doctors told her. She shared her feelings with the social worker. Although she was discharged once for a few days, she spent most of her time in the hospital. She died four months after her diagnosis.

During those four months, the social worker visited Mrs. K. in the hospital on a daily basis, often two or three times during the day. The social worker arranged for the Social Security office to send a representative to the hospital to begin disability coverage and to be certain the children would receive benefits if Mrs. K. died. The social worker managed to get CHAMPUS coverage, which is insurance for federal employees and their family members, extended to the two youngest children and assisted Mrs. K. with all the forms needed to accomplish these tasks. Such concrete services allowed Mrs. K. to take the time to reminisce with the social worker. Mrs. K. was able to resolve problems with some of her older children and to sort out, with the social worker's help, what she wanted for her younger children after she died.

What are the similarities between Mr. F. and Mrs. K.? What are dissimilarities? They were both terminally ill. Mr. F. endured more than two years of the chronic living-dying phase and only approximately five weeks of the terminal phase; Mrs. K. experienced a brief, chronic living-dying experience of about a month and a three-month period of being in a terminal phase. After the first month, Mrs. K. experienced almost constant pain, regular vomiting, inability to eat, constipation, and general malaise. Her body wasted away during the terminal phase. Mr. F. never experienced chronic pain or vomiting but had sleep disturbances and constipation and woke up at night feeling unable to breathe. In the last few weeks he ate very little.

These particular patients provide examples of the basic needs of many patients. Each one is different, but all need support, caring, family or loved ones, tasks completed, and help in coping with the dying experience. The social worker provides concrete services, listens to symptom complaints and helps to resolve them if possible, and enables patients to reminisce, to complete tasks, and to come to terms with the dying experience in whatever way possible.

A most interesting comment from Mr. F. early in his time with the social worker was, "I keep a night-light on like a small child when I go to sleep." Her response was that severe illness makes us like children in some ways. He said, "I'm afraid if I die at night, I won't be able to see what it's like!" The social worker shared with Mr. and Mrs. F. that the night-light seemed likely a symbolic means of keeping death at bay. Kastenbaum and Aisenberg (1976, p. 48) note that we do not wish to be alive when we die, that we attempt to block out the image of the final scene.

Mrs. K. had much less time than Mr. F. to work through the myriad feelings created by her dying. She focused on minutiae such as the dress she wanted to be buried in. She called her surgeon the "crepe hanger" and her internist the "smiler." The surgeon would come into her room and complain that he could not locate the primary site of her cancer and always looked downcast. Her internist would enter her room each day with a smile and say, "We look well today." The social worker had been present many times when the surgeon or internist visited Mrs. K. and listened to Mrs. K.'s description appreciatively. Then Mrs. K. began to focus on her symptoms; they were distressing and all-consuming. Mrs. K. shared with the social worker that she hated vomiting, and yet it was occurring constantly. The definition of terminal illness includes the patient's view of her physician's need to hide from her the occurrence of her overwhelming distress of symptoms.

Pain and Symptom Relief

The social worker took time to discuss these symptoms, as well as Mrs. K.'s pain, with the consulting hematologist. It was 1978, and current methods of pain and symptom control still were not an accepted part of the treatment of terminally ill patients. Yet the hematologist agreed to begin a Brompton's cocktail (an analgesic mixture, often containing morphine and Compazine or a phenothiazine), which relieved pain and nausea to some extent. Twycross (1975, p. 15), who discusses many types of pain medication, suggests pain is a psychological phenomenon, and "chronic pain differs from acute pain in that it is a situation rather than an event, impossible to predict when it will end, usually gets worse rather than better, appears to be entirely meaningless, and frequently expands to occupy the patient's whole attention, isolating him from the world around." This description is as true today as it was twenty-five years ago.

This is an excellent description of the situation that Mrs. K. confronted. The vomiting and pain were unending, and they caused personality aberrations and total absorption by the patient. The worker often held Mrs. K. in her arms. Pain can be overwhelming, and the social worker's response is to be empathetic, to listen to the patient's complaints, and to discuss with the physician and nursing staff how to treat the patient's pain. They can often make a joint decision on how best to help the patient with pain.

Patient and family both have the right to expect the patient's symptoms to be carefully and thoroughly controlled. Each symptom should be treated separately. Symptom control includes emotional, financial, social, and spiritual help, as well as pain control and physical comfort. However, an additional comment about pain and terminal illness is germane: "Pain is a psychological phenomenon, that is, apart from anatomical and physiological components, it has a psychological aspect" (Twycross, 1975, p. 15). Pain thresholds vary biologically and subjectively. Drug studies in hospices have shown that after a patient has begun a course of analgesic relief, heroin or morphine, the needed dose goes down (Berry and Ward, 1995). Pain relief is believed to be accomplished by both medication and emotional support. Twycross comments that when the doctor-patient relationship improves, the dosage can be reduced. He also states that it is theoretically possible to relieve pain in every case of the 40 percent of cancer patients who experience pain. When physical pain is controlled, the pain then experienced is psychosocial, including feelings of displacement, dependency, helplessness, loss of control, fear of the unknown, and fear of abandonment.

The fear of dying is often associated with the fear of pain. The pain related to dying has become a political problem in California and Oregon, where, in 1996, voters approved initiatives legalizing marijuana for medical needs. Marijuana reduces nausea and helps ease pain. Physician-assisted suicide is another political issue, and a referendum in Oregon to legalize assisted suicide was passed in 1994. It is still tied up in the courts. However, in states around the country, signatures are being collected both for the legal use of marijuana for medical purposes and for assisted suicide.

Despite beliefs about pain, it is not a universal experience for the dying. Doyle, Hanks, and MacDonald (1993) stated that in 500 deaths, ninety suffered bodily pain. The great majority gave no signs one way or the other. Their death was similar to going to sleep and forgetting. Perhaps the perception of pain is associated with fear of the unknown. Another survey reported by Fackelmann (1999) states that by more than a 2:1 ratio, Americans say that, rather than focus on making assisted suicide legal, the nation should make pain relief for dying patients a top priority.

Physical Needs

Still, the social worker always has to keep in mind the concern stated by Lack and Buckingham (1978, p. 91), namely, that service to the dying must include smoothing sheets, rubbing bottoms, and relieving constipation and other discomforts. They comment, "Counseling a person who is lying in a wet bed is ludicrous" (p. 91). Thus, the physical needs of the patient must be met before the worker can help the patient cope emotionally with the illness. Further, the worker must alert other health personnel to physical needs and discuss distressing symptoms and pain with nurses and physicians.

MODELS OF THE DYING PROCESS

Two frameworks denote the terminal phase of illness: one is a conceptual model, the other a clinical model. I will also describe an alternate conceptual model.

The first model, Figure 2.1, consists of three stages: the crisis of knowledge of death, the chronic living-dying phase, and the terminal phase of withdrawal.

If it is possible and the social worker is available during the acute crisis phase (as was the case with Mrs. K.), then there is more opportunity to help the patient during the chronic living-dying process. The interventions can help the patient integrate the dying process into his or her life circumstances and, finally, can assist the patient and caregivers to move into the terminal phase when it becomes appropriate.

The clinical model is depicted by Gonda and Ruark (1984, p. 112), as presented by Chaplain Young at Stanford University Medical Center (1976). It emphasizes a clinically important cross-over point: the juncture at which additional medical therapy ceases to extend living and only prolongs the difficult process of dying.

Figure 2.2 depicts the trajectory of dying. Point A represents birth, X denotes the diagnosis of a life-threatening condition, Y is the point past which medical interventions act to prolong dying rather than living, and Z indicates death.

These figures suggest the problem is one of defining as precisely as possible when the transition from living with a life-threatening illness to being terminally ill takes place. Each of the writers cited confirms the individuality of the patient and the fact that the personality of involved clinicians makes a difference. Their point is that

FIGURE 2.1. Conceptual Model

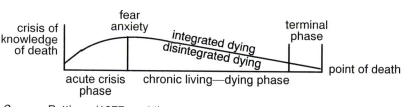

Source: Pattison (1977, p. 44).

FIGURE 2.2. Clinical Model

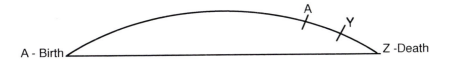

Source: Gonda and Ruark (1984, p. 112).

clinicians who persist with curative attempts and who are heavily invested in those attempts may have difficulty switching from quantity to quality of life as a primary focus.

The two graphic representations of the process of terminal illness provide a sense of how terminal illness is perceived by health personnel who manage patients and their caregivers. An alternate representation can be made by considering the way in which the patient or caregivers perceive the process of the illness. This third model agrees that the point of diagnosis may be one of peak anxiety, or it may be one of denial and minor anxiety. If the illness goes into remission for a period of time, the patient and family may experience relative normality. Then when the illness reoccurs, a peak anxiety may occur, or recur, and subsequently be followed by valleys and peaks of anxiety, depending upon the personality of the patient, family members, and involved clinicians.

As the patient approaches death, as Figure 2.3 suggests, he or she experiences either integration with reduced anxiety and denial or fear with heightened anxiety.

FIGURE 2.3. Additional Conceptual Model

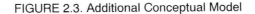
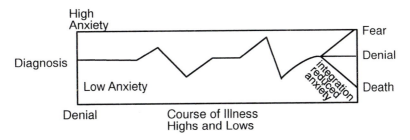

Therefore, emotional reactions of patients and caregivers will follow cycles, usually based on the status of remission and exacerbation of the disease. Often each exacerbation creates new losses and new problems; feelings can become very intense. Fears of the unknown, abandonment, isolation, loss of bodily control, and pain are some of the recurrent characteristics. Such feelings are punctuated with denial, anger, and sadness. The social worker's focus is to help patients express some of these feelings, or at least to accept the person in distress. To help patients, workers must understand the process of terminal illness, the peaks and valleys described, the change in bodily functions, the diminished sense of self, and much of the unstated content. Additionally, the worker must recognize each patient and family member's right to considerate, respectful, and individualized care; relief from pain and unpleasant symptoms; open and complete information concerning diagnosis, treatment, procedures, and prognosis; privacy, discretion, and confidentiality; a safe environment; and the opportunity for their own decision making about care and treatment (Daeffler, 1985). This formulation includes the elements of the ideal model of care presented in Chapter 1.

Encouraging and assisting open communication not only allow for a clear and relevant understanding of the illness but may also permit family members to deal more effectively with the multitude of feelings associated with terminal illness and its repercussions (Vess, Moreland, and Schwebel, 1985). The ability to help patients and families feel in control of a largely uncontrollable situation occurs when flexibility is part of the care and treatment plan.

Additionally, the social worker must be aware of the institutional culture in which he or she works and must be able to assess if, in the usual cure orientation of the acute care hospital, there is room to provide time and care to terminally ill patients. Is there a team effort to provide fuller resources to patient, family, and health team members? If members of the health team fail to respond to patients' and caregivers' needs for support, information, autonomy, and understanding, then patients will be forced to accommodate to the institutional norms and die without causing problems. Munley (1983, p. 16) states that the biomedical mode's orientation toward cure is a factor in the tendency of nurses and others to distance themselves from their dying patients. The distancing is a result of ignorance on the part of health workers, including social workers.

THEORETICAL FRAMEWORK
FOR WORKING WITH DYING PATIENTS

"The task of defining death is not a trivial exercise in coining the meaning of a term. Rather, it is an attempt to reach an understanding of the philosophical nature of man and that which is essentially significant to man which is lost at the time of death" (Veatch, 1972, p. 13).

With Veatch's definition in mind, we can examine the several concepts that make up the body of knowledge necessary for work with dying patients.

The Process

First, the social worker is engaged in a process of working through the life task of dying with patients and their significant others. It is important to remember that terminal illness is a process, not an event. Crisis intervention is not useful because the working through begins after the crisis is past.

Cumulative Loss

The concept of cumulative loss is crucial to work with dying patients. Life and growth are composed of a series of losses. A toddler loses babyhood, an adolescent loses childhood, an older adult loses youth, and so on. One can lose material things through forgetfulness, robbery, fire, sale, etc. One can lose parts of the body by amputation, surgery, accident, etc. One can lose jobs, friends, colleagues, and relatives—not always by death, but by moving away, by loss of contact, and by anger. Thus, loss is a cumulative experience. When the social worker begins to work with a terminally ill patient, unless the patient is a baby, he or she already has experienced some losses. Terminally ill patients also are facing the loss of their future and all those persons in their present and future who are or could be important to them.

Denial

It is vital to understand that the concept of denial is a healing potion to the terminally ill. As indicated earlier, denial reduces anxiety, and it also allows the patient and the family to cope with the inundation of changes that are suddenly part of their lives. The advent of terminal illness is an unplanned and unexpected experience. Denial is necessary to help with the multifaceted problems arising when the patient and family go through the process of terminal illness.

Social Work Principles

The basic social work principles—starting where the client is, partializing, focusing, developing trust, and giving credence to the worth, dignity, and integrity of the individual—are part of the interventive armamentarium of the worker with the terminally ill. The working agreement or contract with the dying person is, by nature of the problem, in constant negotiation.

Mrs. S., sixty-seven years old, had advanced breast cancer and was in the hospital for the third time within six months. The worker knew Mrs. S. had experienced the loss of a breast and now was close to the loss of life. She had previously shared that she was worried about her husband: How would he manage without her? She had had a mastectomy eighteen months earlier, and cobalt treatment, but now was dying. The worker held the patient in her arms and let her cry. This was the working agreement. Mrs. S. was frightened, and the physical contact was what she needed. Words were not necessary.

Mr. B., forty-nine years old, had advanced emphysema and was hospitalized for bronchial spasms every couple of months during the last year of his life. The worker visited him in the hospital and in his home. The worker knew he had lost his mobility; he was confined to an oxygen supply. The working agreement was to help Mr. B. with the disabling nature of his illness and to help his wife and five children understand the nature of his illness, the constraints, the special needs, and the constant threat of death.

Both Mrs. S. and Mr. B. died without any resolution or working through of the tasks for themselves or their family members. Both, however, expressed concerns about their family members.

The cases cited illustrate how the theoretical model applies in situations of nonresolution. The working agreement was operant in both cases and included denial and the inability to express the feelings created by the dying experience. In many instances of terminal illness, the dying patient never moves beyond anger, denial, or fear. However, Glaser and Strauss (1966) state that the presence of close relatives and concerned persons does avert feelings of abandonment and is reported by patients as helpful, despite mutual verbal avoidance of important concerns. In those situations in which dying patients cannot share their feelings, they often recognize the stresses to their family members and loved ones. Conversely, family members who are unable to share their feelings may also recognize the stress this silence creates for the patient.

It is crucial to understand that if a person is terminally ill and has had time to live through the process of dying, then loss is a salient factor. Even if there is no working through, a process has taken place, and, as illustrated by the cases of Mrs. S. and Mr. B., loss is experienced. An elderly person such as Mrs. S. could be losing the opportunity to see future grandchildren or to watch those grandchildren already born grow into adulthood. A person Mr. B.'s age loses the opportunity of seeing his own children grow into adulthood. A dying adolescent is losing the possibility of marriage, children, and a career, as well as parents, siblings, grandparents, and friends.

Social workers who fully understand the concept of loss can intervene in many appropriate ways. If verbal intervention is not appropriate, there is always the time and the need for physical contact, holding the patient's hand or holding the patient in one's arms.

Barton (1977) comments that there is growth potential in any stage of life, but in the dying process, the person increases his or her own perception of nonbeing. Dying is a life stage characterized by growth through the process of letting go and an adaptation to the gradual giving up of life by learning to live with an increasing sense of loss; it is being in direct contact with the ongoing threat of nonexistence.

SUMMARY

Terminal illness is defined within a theoretical model that can include the working-through agreement, a process, denial, and cumulative loss. These factors have been discussed by using case examples, figures, and narrative. Now it is time to move beyond the theoretical underpinning to the work with the different parts of the whole, namely, the interdisciplinary team, the patient and family, and the survivors.

Chapter 3

Working with the Interdisciplinary Team

Miss R. watched fearfully as the surgeon and the social worker approached her bed together. When this fifty-one-year-old woman had been admitted to the hospital two days earlier for a hysterectomy, she had shared with the social worker her fear that she had cancer. Miss R. sensed that if the doctor and social worker came in to see her together, it was a bad omen.

Mrs. C., forty-three years old, was in great pain when she became a patient in the hospice unit, but she remembered meeting the nurse, the doctor, the aide, and the social worker. When her pain was alleviated, all members of the team met with Mrs. C. and told her that she was part of a team, and they would all work together to help her feel more comfortable and to relearn the business of living.

MEMBERS OF THE TEAM

The scenarios for Miss R. and Mrs. C. are very different, yet both include the interdisciplinary team. The team can be composed of two professional health care workers—physician and social worker, nurse and chaplain, social worker and nurse, physician and nurse—and it can evolve as a combination of all disciplines. In fact, the team can include physicians, nurses, social workers, physical and occupational therapists, catering staff, domestic staff, maintenance staff, hairdresser and beautician, chaplain, and volunteers. Corr and Corr (1983) refer to it as the caregiving team, one including all these members.

Patient and Family

Even more important, however, is the notion of patient and family as integral members of the team. This point is stressed particularly by Wilson, Ajemian, and Mount (1978), who describe the Royal Victoria Hospital Palliative Care Service in Montreal. These writers relate that the policy of including patient and family on the interdisciplinary team tends to counter the institutional depersonalization many dying patients experience. They go on to say that the inclusion of the patient and family on the health care team requires patience and a clear understanding of goals. This point of view is such a major departure from the usual training of professionals that frequent refocusing on this issue is required during staff meetings (Wilson, Ajemian, and Mount, 1978).

Social work has always begun by affirming the crucial meaning of family for all clients. The family as the basic unit of our society is also the unit of health and should, therefore, be the unit of treatment. Social workers who work with the patient and family as a unit can help to maintain their sense of competence in the face of severe stress. The patient and the family are part of the team. A dying patient represents a stressor event in terms of family crises, and professional services will make their greatest contribution if they are made with the total family context in mind (Hill, 1967, p. 265). The patient and family can contribute needed input to the whole team.

Another stressor that is akin to death is Alzheimer's disease. The expectation for the twenty-first century is that the incidence of 4 million will increase to 17 million. The patients and families who provide care to their loved ones bear not only the financial brunt of the illness but also the psychological and social stresses associated with the burdens of care (Weiner, 1999). Many studies have focused on the stressors of caregivers related to caring for spouses with Alzheimer's disease (Harris, 1993; Cairl and Kosberg, 1993).

The Nurse

Since hospice is primarily a nursing function, nurses are core members of the health team. Raven (1985) states that nurses have an important role in clinical oncology. Nursing care focuses on pain and other symptomatic problems. Nurses monitor the patient's condition and report the patient's status to the physician. The nurse teaches the patient and family how to care for and treat symptoms. In addition, nurses in hospices supervise home health aides and provide ongoing assessments of the patient's condition (Proffitt, 1985).

The patient's referring physician is responsible for medical direction of patient care and treatment. The physician orders all medical treatment and prescribes medication. A major difficulty for physicians has been the formation of dependency relationships with patients, and dying patients can make physicians fearful and anxious, with a wish to separate themselves from their patients (Levine, 1985). Blacher (1987) points out that it is very difficult for the physician who has a series of dying patients to feel fully with them and not be devastated emotionally. This aversion of the physician to the process of dying must be overcome if the physician is to help the patient deal openly with the social, emotional, and spiritual issues surrounding death and then become a working member of the health team.

One physician who understands the team is Flexner (1977, p. 182), who discusses how he used to feel when he, as the physician who was the dominant member of the team, realized he was the professional who spends the least time with the patient and family. He describes a classic caring situation with the doctor in the center and all other health professionals surrounding him, and the patient, friends, and family outside both circles (Figure 3.1). Flexner then depicts his conception of the ideal caring situation, with the patient in the inner circle, the family circling the patient, and health professionals outside, as depicted in Figure 3.2. He comments, "We all must care for the patients' needs together" (p. 182).

As we return to the professionals who are responsible for Miss R.'s care—the hematologist, nurse, and social worker—they meet at the nurses' station to discuss the status of Miss R. When her surgery was performed, they found that the cancer had spread. The admitting surgeon informed Miss R. that he removed a tumor when he performed the surgery and had called in the hematologist as a consultant. She was not directly informed of the cancer diagnosis. Tumor is often a code word for cancer. He told her that after she recovered from surgery, her care would be provided by her internist and hematologist.

The social worker reported that Miss R. was denying the reality of cancer despite her initial fears when she was admitted. The nurse said Miss R. was focused on the postsurgery distress of gas pains

FIGURE 3.1. Classical Caring Situation

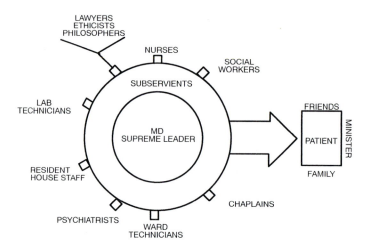

Source: Flexner (1977).

FIGURE 3.2. Ideal Caring Situation

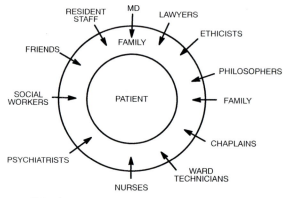

Source: Flexner (1977).

and unhappiness with the IV (intravenous) tube in her arm, the nasogastric tube down her throat, and the hours or days until their removal. The hematologist said that medical treatment would be deferred until after hospital discharge. There was minimal exchange—only a reporting of information. No feedback came from the nonphysician professionals. Perhaps the physician had heard from the nurse and social worker that the patient was not emotionally ready for treatment, or perhaps he felt that the patient was not physically ready for treatment.

The individuals described here do not constitute a team, but a collection of professionals sharing information about a patient without making plans for the ongoing care of the patient. The doctor for Miss R. did not give orders, but it has been noted that physician communication in teams frequently is oriented toward giving orders, while members with lower occupational status convey information (Feiger and Schmitt, 1979).

The surgeon and the internist could have been members of Miss R.'s team, as could the involved family members. But the domain of each is rigidly demarcated in the acute care hospital setting, and the inclusion of family members with the health team is not part of "professional practice." Either the physician alone, the nurse alone, or the social worker alone talks to the family. The social worker, however, could have asked the hematologist to elaborate on his thinking, or perhaps the social worker might have asked for a plan of management for Miss R. during her remaining days as a hospital patient. Such an action would have involved the nurse with the ongoing process and assisted the social worker with discharge and home care plans. Clearly, interdisciplinary team practice in the acute care hospital is still evolving. Currently, team practice is more accepted and works more toward patient needs.

The Relationship Between Nurse and Physician

It is important for social workers to understand the relationship between physicians and nurses. It is suggested that a natural schism exists between physicians and nurses because of the differences in goals, training, technology, attitudes, and population composition of the two groups. There is also a difference in status. The relative disparity between both status and income in an assumed egalitarian society implies many conflicts between nurse and physician. Also, although the physician spends the least time with the patient and the nurse spends the most time with the patient, the physician assumes a leadership role among the health professionals. These factors affect nurses' feelings and can serve as obstacles to effective health team practice (Peeples and Francis, 1968). This condition has not changed greatly in recent years.

Social Workers

Social workers in health settings would do well to learn the nurse orientation to patients. Social workers are considered auxiliary in skilled nursing facilities and home care agencies. Social work services are used to provide social assessments on paper and to provide supervision to non-MSW workers who may be on the site. In these agencies, social workers can use their liaison skills to help develop interdisciplinary teams to provide more comprehensive services to dying patients and their families.

Social workers also provide counseling and guidance to the patient and family in all settings. In hospices, social workers make home visits and provide community resources as needed. Social workers also do staff development counseling. The social worker perceives the social context of dying patients and families and understands the environmental concerns. The social worker has been regarded in many settings as a key member of an interdisciplinary health care team (Goldberg and Tull, 1983).

Social workers on a team are aware that if every team member feels that no one person has all the answers in caring for the dying patient and the family, the effort is likely to be cooperative, involving social worker, physician, nurse, patient, family, and other members of the team. The physicians in these situations are no longer in the position of the all-knowing leader.

ORIGINS OF THE INTERDISCIPLINARY TEAM CONCEPT

The Mental Health Team

The modern health care interdisciplinary team has grown out of the mental health model. The community mental health movement produced a body of literature related to team practice beginning in the middle 1960s (New, 1965, 1968; Rodman and Kolodny, 1965).

The team in the mental health setting usually consists of a psychiatrist, psychologist, social worker, and family worker (paraprofessional). Although team practice was incorporated into the jargon of mental health practice, it was not always put into use. For the team to work, it was important for all disciplines to have a similar philosophy about treatment. In some settings, the psychiatrist in charge could favor a treatment modality that focused on the dynamics of the individual rather than on the social root of mental illness. The fact that a setting has a team, whether it is a community mental health program or a hospital ward, does not mean that professionals are working together to better serve their clients. This is the rhetoric often used for organizing a team. A complete understanding of one another's functions and respect for one another must be in place for the client to receive the benefits of team practice. The shortage of trained professionals and the need to involve the community leads to the paraprofessionals taking on the line work and providing most of the direct service. These trends tend to focus the members of the treatment group to work as a team.

An early examination of the mental health team concept suggested six important premises: equality, knowledge, professions, marginality, task, and domain.

Equality

The concept of equality can mean some team members have more power and authority than others. The physician is the only one with the authority to prescribe medications. Competence by itself implies a certain amount of inequality; some persons are more capable than others. It is a difficult concept to operationalize.

Knowledge

The concept of knowledge indicates that a team brings several persons with specialized knowledge together. The assumption is that different persons bring different knowledge, which is shared for the benefit of improved service to clients.

Professions

If the team members come from different professions, then each one may be very specialized, which requires many professionals to tackle one problem. The professional background may create tension between narrow specialization and a generalist approach to problem solving.

Marginality

Some professions have been established for a long period of time and others are just beginning. Such disparity can result in the marginality of certain professions. This is related to the problem of equality and can interfere with teamwork because members get caught up with status, prestige, and power issues.

Task

If the assumption is that team members work for the common good, then should the boundaries of individuals' tasks be permeable? Some task delineations could be specific, but the ability to do one another's tasks when necessary should be part of team practice. New (1968, p. 324) states, "In teamwork, maybe the rule is fluidity of boundaries yet recognition at all times that each person does have his sphere of talent." This idea helps teamwork fit into any system and bypasses the problem of role blurring.

Domain

Our domain is the area of expertise or responsibility we claim. This is the overriding assumption. It will hinder teamwork if the members claim their domains without sharing, and help teamwork if members claim their domains as a cooperative effort for the common good.

Milieu Therapy

The ideas on the therapeutic milieu, put forth in the early 1960s, were very influential in a movement toward teamwork. Therapeutic milieu meant the whole institution operated as a total community. All interventions with clients were considered a part of the therapeutic community. In the early days, clients were in settings for longer stays and were easier to handle. Today, because of laws, only the most dangerous clients are hospitalized. The nature of milieu therapy, as originally conceived, is such that teamwork becomes a necessity. When the entire institutional setting is part of the therapy, then it becomes most important for the helping disciplines to be coordinated in their efforts to serve the patients. Milieu therapy was widely accepted in the early days of the mental health arena. In fact, there was such a swing from the hierarchical model to the milieu therapy model that professional roles tended to blur. Germain (1984, pp. 198-199) comments that, although the community mental health movement strengthened the team concept, such interdisciplinary team practice in mental health settings led to role blurring, role fusion, and ambiguity of function and task, which served to weaken the team.

The anonymity of team membership can give tacit permission to behave in less responsible ways because group appraisal is not as severe as self-appraisal. Also, teams, similar to institutions, may provide a protective covering for the members to hide under, reducing the likelihood of more direct communication with patients. In effect, training in teamwork can guarantee that trainees will never be left to their own devices and that they will never be urgently forced to become self-aware or to face their own feelings and inadequacies. In effect, "If egalitarian teamwork brings about sufficient blurring of roles and if jobs are sufficiently undifferentiated, the full thrust of each member's clinical effectiveness is never felt" (Rae-Grant and Marcuse, 1968, p. 5).

Rae-Grant and Marcuse were correct to alert professionals not to consider the concept of teamwork a panacea for many of the problems of the evolving mental health system. The sensible conclusion was that teamwork was not toxic, but it also was not the miracle cure.

INTRODUCTION OF THE TEAM CONCEPT
TO THE ACUTE CARE HOSPITAL

Holistic Approach

The concept of the team moved into the physical health arena in the late 1960s and early 1970s. The concepts from the mental health movement were, at times, transferred intact to the acute care hospital. Williams et al. (1970, pp. 957-961) discuss the use of a therapeutic milieu on a continuing care unit of a general hospital. The major effort of the continuing care unit was to move a person from the "sick" role to the well role. The unit provided patient group meetings, specific disease groups, patient/staff meetings, group physical therapy, and patient/family/staff meetings. One of the end results, in addition to helping patients become well in holistic ways, which means the ability to see the patient as a person in a social situation, was to teach medical students, resident physicians, and private physicians that the patient is more than a person dominated by an illness but a whole person whose personhood affects the course of sickness and health. It should be observed that such an arrangement of a continuing care unit in today's acute care hospital is not likely to exist. The DRG (diagnosis-related group) discharge planning mandate of the reimbursement structure does not allow for consideration of the whole person, only the medical diagnosis-related group.

The pressure of the discharge system can be illustrated by what happened to an elderly couple in California in 1983. The husband, in his middle seventies, developed a brain tumor that was treated on an outpatient basis. He was admitted to the hospital for minor surgery and experienced a major stroke while in the recovery room. He moved in and out of consciousness for nine days in the acute care hospital. On the tenth day he was discharged to a skilled nursing facility despite the wife's vociferous protests. He died less than twelve hours following the transfer to the nursing home. He was obviously dying, and the need for discharge from the hospital disregarded both the patient and his wife and attended only to the hospital's need. Reamer (1985) comments that the vast majority of hospital staff do their best to ensure that patients are not discharged prematurely, although such discharges may occur more frequently in cases in which a patient's illness falls into a DRG category that involves less profitable or more costly treatment. It is clear that dying patients are not acceptable DRG patients. Dyer (1986) comments that the issue of cost is now an inescapable part of medical practice.

Rehabilitation Medical Care As a Team Concept

One model of team practice in the health care arena has a long and venerable history. Rehabilitation as a team concept appeared following World War II due to a concern for disabled veterans. Germain (1984, p. 198) states that rehabilitation teams were coordinated by a physiatrist (a specialist in physical medicine). She notes that in the rehabilitation team, recognition of the contributions that could be made by several disciplines working together was present, but the principles evolved rapidly, and the rehabilitation team came to represent a special service in the acute care setting. As indicated, rehabilitation teams are coordinated by a physiatrist and usually include physical therapists, an occupational therapist, a speech therapist, rehabilitation nurses, and a social worker. Team members meet on a weekly basis to discuss the treatment needs of patients in a group. Each discipline contributes to the treatment plan, and attention is paid to psychosocial as well as organic needs.

In 1978, a study of a rehabilitation interdisciplinary team was conducted in a large urban hospital. The study was based on the assumption that if the team is able to function smoothly as a group, then the patients will naturally receive better services. The purpose of the study was to assess the effectiveness of a rehabilitation team in achieving functional health in the care of stroke patients. This particular team included a rehabilitation nurse, physical therapist, occupational therapist, pharmacist, dietitian, speech pathologist, social worker, chaplain, and two physiatrists. Functional health is a multifaceted concept, and team efforts were directed toward the physical, psychological, educational, spiritual, social, and vocational rehabilitation of the patient. Twenty-six patients referred to the team over a seven-month period were compared to thirty-two patients not referred to the team. The results indicate that patients seen by the team scored higher on functional health than those not seen by the team (Pendarvis and Grinnel, 1980).

Members of rehabilitation teams in acute care hospitals often work with terminally ill patients. Patients with metastatic bone disease benefit from occupational and physical therapy geared to their limitations. A person with such a disease can experience extraordinary pain if the bed coverings are moved and can break bones if turned incorrectly. Team members can assist floor nurses who have no rehabilitation training with specific needs of patients with bone and lung cancer.

A sixty-six-year-old man with lung cancer is a case in point. The rehabilitation team was teaching him to breathe and ambulate in ways that would reduce pain and provide limited mobility. The team was prepared to discharge him home with a weekly physical therapy visit and visiting nurse contacts when the social worker informed the team that the patient had a spouse at home who was confined to a wheelchair from a stroke. During his hospitalization, family members had been meeting her needs, but the family felt both husband and wife needed placement in a skilled nursing facility. The husband, however, was adamantly opposed. This information changed the discharge plan, which was delayed for a few days until an eight-hour-a-day home health aide could be sent to the home and a referral made to a local hospice. The rehabilitation team fought for the extra days. This plan of action allowed two alert adults to continue to live in their own home. Although they were physically impaired, they could manage with a home health aide and family backup.

Another example of an interdisciplinary care team provides a different view. Kustoborder (1980) describes an interdisciplinary team in a ninety-eight-bed separate section of an 850-bed hospital. This special section provides extra time for patients who need rehabilitation, recuperation, or terminal care. The team consists of a social worker, a gerontological clinical specialist, a nursing supervisor, a pharmacist, a dietitian, physical therapists, and occupational therapists. The team was examining discharge problems for high-risk patients. Admission reviews were done by the team, and each member learned more about the other team members; this, in turn, promoted coordinated care for the patient and family. Physicians were contacted more frequently for desired orders as a result of team meetings, and nurses were more confident when requesting orders. If the nurse indicated the patient was nauseated, if the dietitian said the patient was not eating, and if the physical therapist found the patient too weak for exercise, the pharmacist was better able to recommend medication. If the social worker contributed information obtained from families on confused patients' previous food habits, preferences, and meal patterns, the dietitian was better able to plan meals to stimulate patients' appetites. The physical and occupational therapists worked with the dietitian with patients unable to swallow, and the occupational therapist advised the dietitian and nursing staff on methods and utensils to encourage independent eating.

Team members reported that their meetings helped them to identify problems early. They learned more about each patient than they would have learned individually, and a general feeling of camaraderie developed as team members learned about one another's roles. The team assumed patient care improved because more patients were discharged to home than to long-term care facilities (Kustoborder, 1980). This type of team may be constrained in today's cost-conscious DRG climate, but it can continue to operate, provided staff can discharge patients within given lengths of stay.

How an Interdisciplinary Team Works

The major focus of the team interaction consists of sharing varying perspectives and sets of information about the patient, the definition of the health problem, and the determination of a health care plan through a process of problem solving.

Nurses from home care agencies take care of some of the most isolated dying patients. They see elderly persons with cancer, emphysema, and coronary disease who are all alone. Some patients have family members who are always present, which may mean the family member is also isolated. The nurse is the most frequent visitor and is responsible for referral to the social worker if the agency has a social worker on staff. These agencies have staff meetings but do not engage in interdisciplinary team practice.

Brill (1976) suggests one of the problems of team meetings is that they are often more time-consuming for busy specialists than are consultation and referral outside the team framework. If the social worker attends the staff meetings of the home care agency and is working with the dying patient, she or he can suggest working as a team. The social worker can try to make it clear that the assets of teamwork include not only an increase in the effective use of specialized knowledge but also a more comprehensive, integrated range of services that provides more complete service to patients and families.

Many social workers in acute care hospitals and skilled nursing facilities develop teamwork with nurses, although the doctors are more elusive. One social worker reported such a set of circumstances in a hospital when the doctor requested, "Please speak to this patient." The doctor had given the patient the bad news of the diagnosis. The social worker said, "Most doctors don't ask for me in cases like this—it depends on physician sensitivity—so my contact with dying patients is limited. However, I provide group sessions to the nurses when they tell me on rounds, 'I can't take it anymore.' "

One of the lessons learned at the hospice is that the end-of-life choice is hard to make. There is so much silence to dying. We are not schooled in end-of-life planning or saying good-bye. If there is time as a patient approaches the end of life, it is better if such sentiments are openly discussed among family members and the patient. As physicians begin to understand the hospice concept, they can become an integral part of the hospice team.

The director of social work of a large skilled nursing facility in the New York metropolitan area reported the following experience:

> One night a woman was dying, and her daughter was with her. I was able to help facilitate the daughter's being able to talk to her mother, even though her mother was comatose. She said, "There's so much I want to say to my mother." I said, "Go ahead, your mother can hear you; watch her eyes flicker." The daughter began talking, and it brought tears to my eyes. I was holding the patient's hand and the daughter's hand. She told her mother what she felt bad about, how much she loved her, and how much she wanted her mother to know it. Shortly after, her mother died. It was sad and exhausting for me, but after the daughter left, I found the supervising nurse and told her about it and felt better.

This case is an example of the social worker doing a very important piece of work, but doing it alone. The worker, however, later involved the nurse to help her process her feelings. This particular nursing facility had regular staff meetings that included all staff:

nursing, social work, dietary, medical records, and the chaplain. The doctors did not attend, and the physical therapist came only if patients being discussed were receiving therapy. The team only discussed dying patients incidentally, which is true in skilled nursing homes and home care agencies.

When talking with a nurse and social worker together at an acute care hospital, the nurse reported that when working with terminally ill patients, the team approach was missing, focus on family was missing, and volunteer assistance was missing. The social worker remarked, "We share the work. M. works with pain. I get the family away from the floor and the patient to take the heat off the situation. I work with patients also, and help the nurses." In this hospital, although the nurse complained about the lack of a team, the social worker and nurse were, in fact, a strong working team.

Social work is more advanced in the area of interpersonal relationships, and, thus, social workers can often see what team colleagues may lack. Social workers also are able to assess the values and strengths of teamwork when health professionals are involved with dying patients and families. If the physician asks the social worker to see a patient to whom he or she has given a diagnosis of a life-threatening illness, the social worker should seek out the physician after contact with the patient and suggest a team meeting between physician, nurse, and social worker to develop a coherent treatment plan, including the medical and psychosocial needs of the patient. When rapport is good between nursing and social work, social workers and nurses should try to involve primary care physicians in achieving more complete services for dying patients and families. The social worker's familiarity with the group process can be an important factor in facilitating team interaction and communication (Lee, 1980).

A social worker at another acute care hospital reported working with a twenty-one-year-old man who had Hodgkin's disease but was vibrant and active. She saw him for several admissions over a period of two and a half years. When the disease was in stage four (the most advanced stage), he was admitted to the hospital with a limited time to live. The worker said, "He knows and you know he's dying. It's very stressful and requires everyone to work together— the primary nurse, the oncology coordinator nurse, the social worker, and the patient." She continued, "We let the patient be his own decision maker on who he wanted to see on the team."

This social worker went on to say that if the physician and nurse support the social worker, it is much easier to work as a team. She said that the oncology coordinator nurse had developed a team to discuss terminal illness, cancer, and management of patients. The team included the coordinator, dietitian, social worker, utilization review nurse, and the IV nurse. One can assume this particular hospital supports the time and care given to dying patients by staff, since a nurse was hired to coordinate services. This is support of nurses who provide much of the hands-on service, and nurses involve dietitians and social workers to provide the other necessary services.

In most hospitals, the care for dying patients tends to be ad hoc. Social workers frequently are trying to coordinate the needs of the dying patient, and a lot of time is spent in individual meetings with members of different disciplines.

Another task the social worker can assume is to develop an oncology team in an acute care hospital. It may not always result in the hiring of an oncology coordinator, but if it results in better working conditions, then team members can provide better care to dying patients and their families. The social worker can work to develop a strong relationship with the supervising nurse, and together they can bring about changes that benefit the staff and the patients. In cooperation with the nursing supervisor, a memo can be sent to all appropriate disciplines, including the primary physician, giving a time and place to meet together to discuss the needs of the dying patients. If three disciplines can come together, it is a start in the right direction. The dying patient has so many needs—pain and symptom relief, diet, mobility, family concerns, spiritual needs, undone tasks, financial concerns, medical needs, feelings, etc.—that no one discipline can begin to meet them all.

A beginning attempt to develop a team in a primary care setting is discussed by Lee (1980). It began as a rigid system in which new data were supplied by team members to the physician, who made all the final decisions. This model shifted, with experience, to one in which the primary decision maker was determined by the decisions that had to be made. Thus, if the particular problem was primarily nutritional, it could be the nutritionist who orchestrated the final decision. This team evolved over time into a working group that struggled with formation, goal selection, role ambiguity, role evaluation, role flexibility, and decision making. These are components of all teams in any health setting. There must be a commitment to team practice before these concepts ever come into play.

THE HOSPITAL INTERDISCIPLINARY TEAM

When the home care agency is compared to the hospice, an interesting phenomenon emerges. This is the phenomenon of site. Hospice care can be found in several locations. A few are in free-standing buildings, most are located in hospital units, and a handful are in skilled nursing facilities. Nonetheless, every hospice program has a large home care component, and some hospice programs are only home care. All hospice programs work together with the local home care/visiting nurse agency.

Hospice care is often defined as home care supplemented by a variety of inpatient services and social services. These services are coordinated by an interdisciplinary team that ideally includes physicians, nurses, social workers, a chaplain, psychologist, dietitian, pharmacist, physiotherapist, and specially trained volunteers (Gray-Toft and Anderson, 1983). The first hospice model in the United States was the Connecticut Hospice, which began as a home care operation and then became a freestanding hospice. The interdisciplinary home care team of the Connecticut Hospice consists of physicians, nurses (RNs and LPNs), a pharmacist, psychiatrist, physical therapist, social worker, volunteer director and volunteers, and secretaries (Lack and Buckingham, 1978).

The Riverside Hospice in Boonton, New Jersey, is a small inpatient house with sixteen beds that carries a census of fifty patients. Usually forty to forty-five of the patients are carried on the home care service. In early 1980, the social worker reported that this hospice employed six home care nurses, four full-time. The full-time nurses could carry up to ten patients. The nurses did at least two visits after death to provide a coping assessment. The social worker was filling in to serve as a bereavement representative. Preparations were underway to hire another social worker to coordinate the bereavement service and be available to provide counseling if needed. The social worker reported that there was no rotation of those working in the inpatient facility and those in home care. She stated that the person in the field was flexible and easygoing, with interviews running longer. The people inside were on schedules, but home care nurses came into the facility to see their patients, and the inside staff called patients when they went home. The team at Riverside included a nursing director, social worker, health educator, director of volunteers, physician, clergy, home care nurses, and one inpatient nurse.

Little has been written or reported about including the patient on the interdisciplinary hospice team. Although hospice philosophy purports to include the patient as a member of the team, that notion has not been examined in a scholarly manner. Some ad hoc incidents have been reported about patients being included on the hospice team and statements about what ought to be done, but there is no rigorous examination. Every description of hospice reports, in detail, the makeup of the interdisciplinary team, its relationship to patients and families, and the necessity of having such a team to achieve hospice goals.

Viney (1984, p. 153) states that professionals, paraprofessionals, families, and friends who wish to help dying patients need to know more about the patients' concerns about death. The team members also need to know patients' feelings about the care plans being made for them and to be involved with the professionals and other health care personnel in all phases of treatment. The involvement of dying patients on the interdisciplinary team ought to become an area of research so that the findings can help treatment personnel understand the extent to which interdisciplinary teams are compatible with the needs of patients.

Another viewpoint suggests that the idea of the patient as a hospice team member is absolutely wrong. Kane (1982, p. 4) notes that the patient's role with respect to the health team is to define the problem and to use the services and recommendations offered by the team insofar as the latter have value. The patient is the focus of the work, the person who defines the goals, sets priorities, and is the ultimate decision maker. Kane says health care providers should be able to give the needed service pleasantly and expeditiously without subjecting the patient to the hassles of becoming a member of an interdisciplinary team.

These divergent views confirm the need for research that would sort out the meaning of the patient on the team. I suggest that a patient who defines goals, sets priorities, and makes decisions about care and treatment is, in fact, a member of the team. Behind the patient's becoming a member of the team is the notion of empowerment, which is the role ascribed to the patient by Kane. I commented earlier that in more recent literature, the patient and family are considered part of the team.

Characteristics of the Interdisciplinary Team

The interdisciplinary hospice team requires of its members a willingness to learn from one another, as was done at the Connecticut and Riverside hospices, and, within the limits of legal restriction, to cross disciplinary boundaries when that is required for need-oriented care. Corr and Corr (1983) note that a physician making a home visit alone must be willing to clean up vomit, just as a social worker must help a patient to the toilet or a nurse must sit down at the bedside to listen to an urgent sharing from a dying person.

A social worker from the San Francisco Hospice shared a situation that illustrates this concept in operation. She was working with a woman in her middle fifties who had lung cancer. Her daughter came from Lake Tahoe to care for her mother at home. The hospice nurse went to the mother's home to teach the daughter how to do the primary care. A volunteer visited the home to provide respite care to the daughter. The social worker made an evaluation visit and helped with insurance coverage, contacted the Cancer Society for needed equipment, and handled other financial needs. The daughter talked on the phone to all team members. Some weeks after the daughter arrived, the social worker stopped in at the house for a visit and was present at the time of death. The social worker contacted the funeral home, helped the daughter dress the deceased patient, and then attended the memorial service and provided follow-up services to the daughter to help her complete unfinished tasks and dispose of her mother's things.

This case serves as a living example of the flexibility needed of every team member. Also, it indicates that the social worker can provide whatever service is needed at the opportune time. This hospice team consisted of the head nurse, a home health aide, volunteers, a social worker, a family member at times, and five hospice staff. The team often met with members of the visiting nurse association and their social workers. The hospice and the home care agency were affiliated.

This illustrates a team working well together, being involved with family and patient, and a timely response. Koff (1980) makes the point that time is crucial to the dying person and the dying person's caregiver. In addition to providing prompt responses to requests, it is essential that there be sufficient staff to accommodate urgent needs. Staff should be ready to use the resources of family and volunteers to respond in a timely fashion. Koff (1980) notes, "Hospice care should provide a team made up of family members, practitioners in various disciplines, and volunteers who regularly respond to personal needs" (p. 115).

Role Blurring

Often, each member of a hospice team takes on varying roles. Munley (1983) discusses role blurring as a positive aspect of hospice care. She states that the prevalence of role blurring in work and in practice suggests that the community emphasis of a hospice program and the phenomenon of role blurring is vital to the effectiveness of hospice care. It is interesting to note that clarity of roles is stressed by Lister (1982) in his discussion of role training for interdisciplinary teamwork. He states that when there is a lack of agreement as to role expectations, conflict usually occurs in the social system. Lister reports that the process of clarifying professional roles eliminates misinformation and imparts new information. These two opposing views reveal the relatively wide gap between an interdisciplinary team in a hospice setting and an interdisciplinary team in a hospital or other health setting.

HOSPICE AS A SELF-HELP CONCEPT

Munley (1983) equates the hospice team with the self-help movement. She says the collaborative stance of professional hospice personnel toward patients, families, and volunteers is similar to the role of professionals involved with self-help groups. Her ideology on hospice/self-help goes a long way in explaining the fact that she calls the blurring of roles vital to hospice. Self-help groups are committed to self-reliance, informality, and may be antiprofessional. Delineated roles are not part of self-help groups.

Make Today Count, a self-help group, was founded by Orville Kelly, a cancer patient, in the early 1970s. It was essentially concurrent with the hospice development in this country. Make Today Count was developed by cancer patients who felt that their needs were not met by the formal health care system. Hospice was developed by the impetus of health care professionals who felt the needs of dying patients were not met by the health care system.

As hospice evolved, it was joined by the lay community. Usually the lay community consisted of family members who had previously experienced the loss of someone close and felt the situation had been poorly handled. The lay community also could include family members whose dying loved ones were presently being handled badly.

The self-help groups and the hospice committees were composed of people who were discouraged and disgruntled with the health care system. Gartner and Reissman (1984, p. 22) state that Make Today Count included a unique combination of those with cancer, their spouses, their friends, and their caregivers. Munley (1983, p. 312) notes, "Hospice extends the theme of self-empowerment to the circumstances of death." In the context of Munley's vision, the blurring of roles is necessary to carry out the mission of hospice, and, understood in this context, the blurring of roles becomes a strength rather than a weakness of the interdisciplinary team. Thus, a goal may be to bring together the convergent views of what constitutes a vibrant interdisciplinary team. The important question to be kept in mind is whether the needs of the dying patient and family are being served fully by the team.

Despite the present climate of retreating from dying persons, studies in the literature help to inform the practitioner in the health care setting about interdisciplinary team practice. Social work and nursing journals continually update ideas and report on studies. Practitioners can become knowledgeable in the ways in which professional teams assist patients and families to set up treatment plans in hospitals, hospices, and skilled nursing facilities. Teams help patients and families follow through with productive discharge plans and care at home.

SUMMARY

A discussion of team practice in mental health settings, rehabilitation medicine, and interdisciplinary health teams in hospitals and hospices suggests a wide area of practice. Nevertheless, examples from specific hospitals, rehabilitation units, and hospices indicate considerable variability in how interdisciplinary teams are defined and where and how they operate within each program. Several generic concepts are evident, including the importance of the alliance between social workers and nurses. Teams must remain aware of ideals, the reality of the practice, and the need to continue to learn how to improve skills and understanding so that interdisciplinary health teams serve the professionals, the patient, and the family.

Chapter 4

Working with the Patient and Family

The skills needed to work with the dying patient and family are not very different from skills used to intervene with any client system. It is important to be open, accepting, and available. The needs, yearnings, and problems are common to all clients, although some of their needs are particular to an awareness of the impending death. Pilsecker (1975) states that to offer one's skills to help the terminally ill patient and family to deal openly with the hard fact of death and to allow the patient's denial of reality without participating in it are challenging tasks for the social worker.

Often the only thing a loved one can do in the face of a dying person's anger or depression is to accept whatever feelings the dying person has, without trying to fix things or cheer the person up (Di-Giulio and Krantz, 1995). In fact, a loved one beginning to accept the reality of the coming of death can assist the dying relative to come to acceptance as well.

Other key findings are: half of those polled think the health care system does not always keep dying patients pain free; eight in ten Americans believe the medical system does only a fair job of making sure that patients do not face overwhelming pain problems.

A survey was funded by the Robert Wood Johnson Foundation and included the American Medical Association and the American Cancer Society. The group recommended that if people get enough pain medication to keep them comfortable, they might not turn to assisted suicide. The group also recommended that all Americans fill out an advance directive spelling out the kind of care desired in case of a severely debilitating or life-threatening illness (Fackelmann, 1999). If a loved one is in a severe auto accident or suffers a major stroke, the family needs to be prepared.

We must come to terms with our own mortality whenever we work with terminally ill patients. We imagine what it would be like to die and can only begin to understand after working with dying patients.

THE SOCIAL WORKER

When death is placed within the developmental structure, it becomes a part of life rather than something terrible "out there." That does not mitigate the sadness. Our feelings are real, and we mourn for the patient.

Mrs. D. was an independent, active woman of seventy-four who had worked outside the home and been a widow for many years. When she became ill, she told the social worker in the hospital that her biggest fear was becoming dependent on her children or grandchildren. In time, over several hospital admissions, she developed a strong relationship with the social worker, with whom she reviewed her life. The patient's sons were unable to discuss her illness with her, and she died without any family discussion of how she felt or how they felt.

A social worker in another hospital became involved with Mr. P., an eighteen-year-old leukemia patient who had been referred for home care assessment. The social worker discovered that the family did not allow their son to talk about his illness. The family was also angry because the floor staff did not share with them what was happening to their son. The social worker told the mother that if she could learn to give shots of Demerol her son could go home, and the social worker said, "I will accept full responsibility." The mother learned to give the injections, and a sibling brought the patient directly to the pediatric ward to see his doctor on a weekly basis. A family member called the hospital floor every evening to talk about the young man's status. The patient was admitted overnight periodically to receive transfusions. The family became open, warm, and secure and made extensive use of hospital staff. The patient died a year after the diagnosis, and the social worker was able to help family members with bereavement.

Assessing the Situation

These two examples are presented to delineate and examine the assumption that work with a terminally ill patient means the family is always included as part of the intervention. Even in hospice settings in which the credo is "patient and family as a unit of care," the family is not always accessible. In certain situations, family members are alienated and will rebuff all attempts by health personnel to bring them into contact with the dying patient. Some patients have no family or their family does not live in the area. Patients may be reluctant to call on family or friends who are busy and involved with their own lives. All these scenarios are part of the social work assessment. Social workers know that patients can be part of fragmented families, combined families, reconstituted families, nuclear families, extended families, and multiple families. Koff (1980, p. 35) comments that sometimes a family conflict will interfere with the comfort of the patient, and the focus of care must be on the dying person.

When working with terminally ill patients, it is clearly the intention of the social worker to intervene with the patient and family. This is the purpose where the family is involved and wants to be consulted. As discussed earlier, "family" is used in the broadest sense and is defined as those who provide the primary care for the dying patient; family can be a spouse, parent, child, sibling, aunt, nephew, friend, lover, or whichever person serves as the primary caretaker. Whenever someone serves in the role of primary caregiver, that person should receive the same consideration from the health team as the patient.

Another illness, Alzheimer's disease, is terminal and in many ways suggests early grief and intimate involvement with the caretaker. Alzheimer's disease is the common dementing illness of later life. The disease starts with the loss of intellectual function and gradual development of profound dementia. Most patients are in their sixties, seventies, and eighties, except for a small group who develop the disease in their forties and fifties. The disease significantly reduces life expectancy (Katzman, Hill, and Esh, 1994). As the disease progresses, language difficulties become prominent, beginning with impaired naming, progressing to aphasia, and culminating in mutism.

Psychiatric symptoms, including depression, paranoia, delusions, and visual hallucinations, are common and occur in the early and middle stages of the disease. Behavioral disturbances such as wandering and aggression are more common in the middle and late stages of the disease. Loss of the ability to dress or feed oneself and to perform the activities of daily living occurs in the late stages of the disease. Urinary and fecal incontinence are also part of the late stages of Alzheimer's disease. Seizures may occur in the late stages. Death usually results from sepsis that follows pulmonary or urinary tract infection.

The annual cost of care for Alzheimer's patients is now estimated at almost $100 billion (Weiner, 1999). The patients and family care providers affected by this disease bear not only the financial costs of the illness but also the psychological and social stresses associated with the burdens of care. The physical stress of dressing, feeding, and helping to bathe and toilet the patient is constantly present. In a group of caregivers with which I have been a facilitator, one of the women, who was four feet ten inches tall, often talked about trying to get her six-foot husband off the toilet. Women have reported having to call the fire department or 911 if their spouses fall, because there is no way one usually smaller woman can lift a larger man who is often a dead weight. The loss associated with Alzheimer's is long term because the loss begins before death. This is especially true for older adults, who, in addition to experiencing the loss of their lifetime spouse, are experiencing other losses.

The diagnosis and prognosis create changing systems for the patient and family as well as the professional health care providers, including the social worker. As medical therapies continue to lengthen the survival time of patients with terminal illnesses, the quality of survival and the emotional consequences of the illness and its treatment become more important (Goldberg and Tull, 1983). Some form of social and psychological adjustments must be faced by every patient and family coping with the diagnosis and the prognosis of a terminal illness.

The family or lack thereof is an essential component of the total situation. Multiple external and internal factors affect the patient, the family, and the health team.

The social worker in a hospital setting visits patients in their rooms and works on developing a relationship, takes into account the situation, takes cues from the patients, and provides warmth and caring. If patients wish to talk about their feelings, they will let the worker know. If the patients want answers, they will ask directly. A social worker at a large teaching hospital says, "I always ask the patient, 'What has the doctor told you you have?' or 'What are you in the hospital for?' " The worker says the patient may reply, "I have gallstones, and they're using radiation as a preventive measure." This worker states that sometimes patients do not know that they have a life-threatening illness; other times, patients are told the diagnosis and they deny or repress the knowledge. She says it surfaces with tears, or they talk about death in symbolic terms.

I agree with much of what this social worker has to say, but not that the patients do not know they are very ill. Patients always know, but since denial is a healthy defense, frequently it allows patients to talk about their illness in terms of gallbladder problems or whatever terms are tolerable for them. The diagnosis of cancer, blood disease, coronary disease, kidney failure, and the like are all catastrophic events, and people need time to learn how to cope with myriad experiences. There are mixed feelings, multiple treatments, a drastically changed environment, job concerns, and family problems; every part of life is affected.

It is good practice to ask the patient questions similar to those posed by this worker; i.e., "Why were you admitted to the hospital?" Such a question allows the worker to sense where the patient is in terms of awareness. It is assumed that the social worker has been in communication with the physician and knows what the patient has been told. If a team is in place, then all health personnel involved with the patient will know where the patient is in regard to the illness. Weisman (1972, p. 66) states, "Patients seem to know and not want to know, they often talk as if they did not know and did not want to be reminded of what they have been told."

It is essential for the social worker to hear when patients wish to discuss their feelings about being terminally ill and their concerns over impending death. And although the social worker understands the necessity of denial, the worker must be careful not to allow patients to feel that they must continue the denial. The social worker listens and enables patients to talk about their concerns regarding dying, losing so much, not living to complete life as once expected, etc. The social worker in all settings has to understand what patients know, how aware they are that they are dying, and how family members are handling the situation.

Kastenbaum (1979) notes that once a person is defined as terminally ill, he or she becomes the property of a health care network and is threatened by loss of autonomy and personhood. Almost any hospital patient experiences a loss of autonomy. As a person enters a hospital, the person becomes someone to whom things are done rather than an active person who is doing things. Drew (1987, p. 19) comments, "Autonomy invariably encompasses action as a member of society, as a sexual being, as a personality, as a family member—indeed, action in every aspect of personhood."

Hospital patients give up their right to decide when, where, and what to eat, when to sleep, and where to walk. Their lives are run for them by forces over which they have no control. The sense of loss of autonomy transforms into a feeling of powerlessness. This is compounded for the dying patient, whose loss of autonomy can seem more extreme because of physical deterioration as well as a loss of control.

Groups are another way to gain control over the environment. Dying patients can do well in groups, as can family members of dying patients. In the group, the helpless become the helpers, which can assist them to move from a dependent role to a more interdependent role.

Groups for terminally ill patients and/or family members of terminally ill patients have been organized in varying settings. The best known is the self-help group Make Today Count, begun in the 1970s. A particular chapter of Make Today Count was described from the point of view of researchers who acted as consultants. They helped the group focus and use techniques to help others in group discussions. The stated purposes of these techniques were to reduce feelings of isolation, reduce feelings of being different or abnormal, avoid arguments, and increase tolerance of different points of view. The changes suggested by the researchers increased patient participation in the group from 10 percent to 50 percent, and the ambiance was much more hopeful (Wollert, Knight, and Levy, 1984, pp. 129-137).

It can be helpful to run support groups in hospitals and skilled nursing facilities for persons who are experiencing similar catastrophic illnesses. Such groups are difficult to begin because there is resistance from the health staff. If families of terminally ill patients can meet in groups, then when and if patients leave the institutional setting, the patients can join the group or create self-help groups. Groups such as Make Today Count are usually sponsored by a health professional until they are able to move under their own steam.

The sense of alienation and loss of control can be decreased if patients are given the opportunity to make decisions whenever possible. Self-care and being able to select menus helps the patient regain some control over the environment and the disease. Removing from a patient all opportunity to act independently defeats the good of enabling patients to maximize their remaining time to "live" until they die (Cassileth and Stinnett, 1982).

The Institution

Bureaucracy may affect the relationship between worker and client. Hospitals are treatment centers, research facilities, and teaching institutions. They are also organizations. Organizational goals are concerned with survival, with economics, and with prestige and other goals that are often in conflict with patients' needs, particularly dying patients' needs. The impersonality of the bureaucracy, which is designed to provide fair treatment, may be interpreted by patients as depersonalization.

Bureaucracies, which are organizations designed to operate efficiently and rationally, are run on schedules. Strauss and Glaser (1970) suggest the discrepancy between staff schedules and patients' inner clocks creates a dissonance between senses of time that may increase a patient's growing isolation. Staff in hospitals and skilled nursing facilities operate on "work time" and schedules that are not related to many patients, both dying and recovering. Dying patients are fit into work schedules, as are all other patients (Kamer-man, 1988).

Another aspect of care that affects the patient is the nature of the team, whether hierarchical or egalitarian. The setting can espouse the concept of teamwork, but if the commitment is not supported by the organization, it will not work. The hierarchical model is associ-ated with hospitals in which the physician runs the team. The hospi-tal can shift rewards from hierarchical components to explicit posi-tive recognition of the team delivery model (Lowe and Herranen, 1981, p. 6). If the team is egalitarian, there is cooperation and respect for team members and respect for dying patients.

Social workers need to examine the settings in which they work or are placed. If the setting provides certain specific aids such as reduced patient-staff ratios, flexible vacations, and opportunities for staff to withdraw in critical stress periods, then social workers can ask whether such measures help them provide better services to their dying clients and, in turn, whether clients gain more assistance in working through life/death problems.

The Patient

The work a social worker does with a terminally ill person begins with using the theoretical formulations suggested in Chapter 2. One of the formulations is understanding that terminal illness is a pro-cess. This process begins with an understanding of the person in the situation. Whether the person is in a hospital, a skilled nursing facility, a hospice, or at home, the intervention will change accord-ing to the external circumstances.

The person mobilizes himself or herself to deal with a diagnosis of cancer, end-stage renal disease, severe coronary disease, or any other catastrophic diagnosis by not hearing the diagnosis until he or she is ready to deal with it. As long as the individual does not deny reality for an extended period so that it becomes dysfunctional, the denial works in service of the ego. Denial supports coping abilities. When the individual becomes a patient, denial again helps the per-son to cope with the severe stresses of dialysis or chemotherapy. The social worker needs to understand the benefit of denial when the situation is overwhelming to the person.

Anger is another reaction to terminal illness. At times, anger provides the patient with strength and vitality. Graham (1985, p. 78), a cancer patient, said:

> Healthy anger gives us purpose, challenges us to make new decisions, encourages old ideas; to enroll in the course we've always wanted to take; to embark on the trip we've always wanted to make; to create the journal that is our legacy to our children and grandchildren.

The patient also has an important need for someone to "be there." For example, a social worker in a hospital, assigned to an elderly man in his late eighties, spent much of her time with him just holding his hand. If he felt the need to talk, the worker was available.

The function of the social worker to establish a relationship that respects and meets the needs of a dying person's fears about the fact of his or her illness is important to the social worker's professional status as an integral part of the health team effort to provide care. "Being there" depends heavily on self-awareness and the understanding that one's presence can be more powerful than words. As Barton (1977) comments, the involved caregiver enables the dying person to find meaning and an enduring sense of vitality even while dying.

A social worker in a skilled nursing facility reports that many patients are aware they are dying but do not feel able to talk with their family members about it. Most family members will say, "Oh, you look good. You're fine!" The worker says patients often talk with her about their feelings. She says she does not give them false hopes. This worker is upset because too many of the residents are sent to the hospital to die. She remarks, "This [skilled nursing facility] is their home, and we can do as much for them here as they do at the hospital."

A worker at another skilled nursing facility says she is a shoulder to cry on; she accepts the person who is dying, is aware of how the environment affects the dying resident, and works hard to ensure that the environment responds to the terminally ill person's needs. This worker watches for nonverbal cues and tries to respond to them. She reports that she has respect for the patient's self-knowledge of time of death. Both nursing home workers make a strong point of the need to be available to patients. One worker states, "Being there is the most important thing I have to offer." The concept of someone being present to help terminally ill patients avoid feelings of isolation and abandonment is documented by many scholars (Barton, 1977; Glaser and Strauss, 1968; Feifel, 1977; Goldstein, 1973; Pilsecker, 1975; McDonnell, 1986).

Another patient concern is control of symptoms. Symptom control, although defined by some as only a medical concern, is broadly conceived to include assisting with psychological, material, and spiritual concerns. As a disease progresses, patients can experience bodily disfigurements that, in turn, can result in the alteration of body image, self-concept, and physical functions. This may then complicate pain reduction and require prompt and sensitive attention. Lack (Lack and Buckingham, 1978, p. 91) comments that patients who are relieved of pain, are well nursed, and have a caring person available can be alleviated of the emotional pain more easily.

The quality of the relationship with the patient often is strengthened if the social worker can help the patient to engage in life review. Such review is an essential component of the process if a patient is to come to terms with his or her illness more effectively. Review includes repetition. It is cleansing to repeat the pieces of the illness that were painful: diagnosis, depression, pain, etc. This review and repetition is a crucial part of working through despair and grief. A similar technique has been noted by professionals who provide psychotherapy to terminally ill patients. Schwartz and Karusu (1977, p. 23) note that if the terminally ill person is engaged in psychotherapy, an acceptance, without reservation, of the patient's life story must be present. The therapist must be able to share in the reliving and working through of the dying person's experience.

When working with the terminally ill, social workers must often begin by granting permission to the patient and family to grieve and then to accept their signs of grief. If patients resist grief feelings, social workers may help by speaking of their own past experiences. Because the dying patient can be caught up in refusal, retreat, and withdrawal, the availability of an accepting social worker who is able to tolerate such demanding reactions is crucial. Otherwise the patient is left alone to cope with unresolved feelings (Liu, 1983, p. 9).

The patient's experience of grief, fear, helplessness, and loss of control are all part of terminal illness, and Kastenbaum (1979, p. 204) comments, "It is still an achievement to help a person maintain self-integrity during the terminal part of life."

Another problem for social workers occurs when the patient is comatose, or there is a discussion between family and physician about withholding treatment. A variety of states have resolved these problems through court action. Some hospitals will honor living wills and/or health care directives. The social worker can help locate family members who can confirm or deny the wishes of a patient in a comatose state or in severe situations of total body paralysis, including the inability to speak.

Nancy Cruzan was the first legal case of a patient whose response was limited to grimaces. She was in a car accident in 1983 and suffered anoxia (lack of oxygen) for twelve to fourteen minutes. She was oblivious to her surroundings and had no hope of improvement. Nancy was not terminally ill but could not improve.

The Missouri State Court ruled that the state's interest in life is unqualified. Nancy Cruzan's father appealed, and in December 1989, the U.S. Supreme Court heard arguments in the Cruzan case. The Supreme Court made three points in *Cruzan v. Director, Missouri Department of Health*. The first point was that a person has a right to refuse medical treatment; in the Cruzan case, the court reestablished this right as a liberty interest. The second point is that incompetent patients also retain a right to refuse treatment, with that right to be exercised by a surrogate decision maker. The court made no requirement of an advance directive. The right to refuse medical treatment includes the right to refuse artificially supplied nutrition and hydration. The third point is that the right to refuse medical treatment may be exercised through a living will, durable power of attorney, or other directives.

Within two hours of the ruling, Nancy's family asked the doctor to remove her feeding tube. Nancy's family kept a twenty-four-hour vigil with her until she died on December 26, 1990, twelve days after her feeding tube was removed (Landes, Siegel, and Foster, 1994).

Social workers sharing how they are able to communicate with dying patients, families, and other health staff can help everyone to assess their abilities for dealing with terminal illness. Orcutt (1977, p. 29) notes that opening up communication and the appropriate sharing helps patients and families become more flexible in their interactions and ability to deal realistically with their grief and the added burdens of their lives caused by the illness.

Hostile and Difficult Patients

Some patients can be very difficult. For example, Mr. D., a double amputee, forty-seven years old, had cancer and was hostile. Except for his wife, the rest of his family had abandoned him. The social worker used the time for support of both parties, information giving, and concrete help. When the worker did not turn away to avoid his hostility, Mr. D. gradually began to trust the worker. The counseling was difficult but essential for the patient and his wife.

Mrs. L., a woman in her seventies, was at home with head and neck cancer and a large fulminating tumor. Her husband was prepared to do all he could for her. The patient felt ugly and wanted to withdraw. She came to the day accommodations room for her chemotherapy, and the social worker saw her there. When Mrs. L. saw that the social worker did not recoil from her appearance, the worker was allowed to visit the patient at home. The worker visited twice and maintained phone contact. The wife died in her sleep; the husband called the social worker to inform her of his wife's passing but could not yet cry. A few days later, the social worker was in the supermarket and met the husband. She said, "He took a look at me and cried." Then he came in for follow-up counseling. The husband knew he could trust the worker who had not been repelled by the ugliness of his wife's illness.

Working with hostile patients or patients with the types of disease that present distasteful odors and sights are the most difficult aspects of work with the terminally ill. Levinson (1975, p. 31) suggests that with difficult dying patients, the worker may need to reduce denial, counter withdrawal and apathy, sanction dependency, and combat depression—all within a brief time span. The approach to such patients must be supportive, directive, and educative.

When working with PWAs (persons with AIDS), the problem is very different because PWAs are usually twenty-three to thirty-five years of age. The loss is powerful. It wipes out everything the patient dreamed of having, doing, or being. The plans made for one's life disappear, and this is particularly poignant for PWAs who are usually twenty-three to thirty-five years of age. The changes in the social and psychological status of PWAs are major. Besides enduring physical isolation and many precautions against transmission of HIV, PWAs must contend with social attitudes based on the early association of the disease with homosexuals and drug users. (In fact, the rate of HIV infection is currently highest among young, female, minority heterosexuals.) They develop respiratory disease, cancer, and dementia. In fact, it is estimated that more than half of the persons diagnosed with AIDS will present with central nervous system dysfunction (Buckingham and Van Gorp, 1988). They experience a drastic change in body image, and their sexual lives often come to an abrupt end. McDonnell (1986, p. 228) comments that the implications for the hospice care team are many when working with PWAs. The implications for health personnel in the acute care hospital or in home health agencies are just as numerous and perhaps more difficult because there is less commitment to compassionate care. And today many HIV-infected persons live many years due to new medications.

A diagnosis of cancer or any other terminal disease is overwhelming in itself, but add to it the youth of PWAs, the fact that they are going to die most likely because of their sexual behavior, and, finally, the fact that the disease is infectious. This creates many negative feelings, including guilt, anger, remorse, depression, despair, isolation, and fear of abandonment (McDonnell, 1986). PWAs must also cope with those professionals and nonprofessionals who want to quarantine them and brand them as a terrible scourge. Social workers involved with PWAs who are homosexual need to understand the components of care: the patient, the patient's lover, and the patient's family. The devastation of a terminal illness in a healthy young individual is compounded by the complex reaction of society and some health care workers' refusal to treat or care for PWAs. If the lover and family are supportive, it is easier to connect the PWA to the necessary resources because persons other than the PWA can help. If the PWA is completely alone, then the worker must become an advocate to help the PWA cope with a series of disasters: physical frailty, loss of income, loss of family, fear, etc.

The National Association of Social Workers (NASW) has recognized an informal Social Workers' AIDS Network (SWAN) which was started in New York City in 1982. Social workers have formed small SWAN groups in many other areas of the country (*NASW News,* 1988, p. 9). The groups continued into the 1990s. It suggests that social workers working with PWAs require specialized knowledge, as discussed previously.

Additional important data include the fact that significant others and friends of PWAs are at high risk for AIDS, substance abuse, and suicide, in particular. PWAs are twice as likely to attempt suicide as are other terminally ill persons. Substance abuse abounds in the gay male community. With substance abuse comes a host of problems: lack of communication, instability, other health problems, denial, and avoidance are likely to be prominent even in the absence of a life-threatening illness (Olson, 1988).

Thus, the social worker will need to help PWAs sort out their problems and relationships and make decisions about their willingness to separate from people who are destructive to them. Building a support base often means limiting or eliminating contact with people who attempt to counter healthy communications and treatment. A social worker needs to know that families range in attitude from self-sacrifice to total rejection. If the family is not rejecting, the social worker and the PWA can work together to assist loved ones to make peace and come to some limited acceptance of reality (Olson, 1988).

PWAs have shared with me that compassion and love are what they want from social workers, nurses, physicians, and others. Social workers and other health personnel who come in contact with PWAs who are in fact homosexuals or drug users must come to terms with their own feelings, their own fears, and their own discomfort with homosexuality and/or drug use before they can provide the compassionate care that is so desperately needed by the growing group of PWAs.

Although AIDS was identified in 1981, it was not until 1984 that the agent believed to be responsible for AIDS was identified. It was then named HTLV-III or LAV, now referred to as HIV, human immunodeficiency virus. Testing was developed in 1984 but not available until 1985 when it was licensed by the U.S. Food and Drug Administration (Johnston, 1995).

Before testing, many gay men began searching for early symptoms of illness, as gay men were the first identifiable group of cases. A blemish on the skin was terrifying; a cold or cough was also frightening. "The dread of being the next one to succumb loomed large in the early years of the epidemic, and fear about one's own health was sometimes accompanied by another more excruciating fear: the fear of having infected a lover unknowingly" (Johnston, 1995, p. 34).

According to Johnston (1995), it is common for gay men today to say that anal sex is "unsafe" even when practiced by two HIV-negative persons. Does this, then, reiterate mainstream culture's negative view of same-sex behavior under the guise of public health?

Social workers employed in the field of HIV/AIDS are acutely aware of working in a high-risk occupational environment and are concerned about the possibility of contracting the disease. They are also aware that their spouses, close friends, and others experience anxiety about being infected. Working with AIDS patients also carries a stigma. Empirical support for this view was given by Wiener and Siegel (1990), who surveyed 210 social workers in twelve hospital centers and found 79 percent felt family or friends were, or would be, concerned about their working with AIDS patients. Knowing what precautions to take to prevent infection, and knowing that casual contact with PWAs does not put one at risk can help to alleviate these concerns.

Social workers are unsure how much to share about work-related issues with AIDS patients. Social workers and other health professionals also may invest so much time and effort in their work that they have trouble achieving a balance between time at work and leisure time. Ross (1993) points out that as a result of general work stress, AIDS-related stresses, and home and personal types of stress, many social workers manifest symptoms of chronic stress, or burnout.

Clearly, HIV testing has not entirely done away with the social and psychological problems gay men experienced before testing began. In the gay community today, almost all members have opted for testing because of the new medications available that can keep symptoms at bay for months or years. However, testing divides the community into two parts: those who are infected and those who are not. It is difficult to think of people as toxic, as we might think of alcohol or cigarettes. "If we all begin to recoil from one another, it will be not just the protection of our lives that we ensure but also the death of our souls" (Johnston, 1995, p. 129).

The field of HIV/AIDS is full of unsanctioned and unrecognized grief. Such grief can be defined as the grief that persons experience when they incur a loss that is not, or cannot be, in the face of misconceptions, openly acknowledged, publicly mourned, or socially supported (Cho and Cassidy, 1994).

THE PATIENT AND FAMILY AS A UNIT OF CARE

As we know, when a person becomes a terminally ill patient, every family member has to cope with this event. This is the case whether there is only one support person or several in the immediate circle of the patient. The threat to life creates heightened anxiety in all families, no matter how emotionally healthy or intellectually prepared they are (Whitt et al., 1981-1982, p. 62). Workers in all health settings encounter family members who are relatively open about the terminal illness of a member but who may have difficulty discussing the illness with the patient. Also, some family members may work at protecting the patient from knowledge about the illness. Usually this results in game playing in which the family behaves as if everything is normal, and the patient participates by acting as if there is no problem. The social worker must relate to each person individually and, hopefully, help each one to explore why he or she needs to play games.

Miss C., fifty-two years old, was admitted to the hospital with a diagnosis of uterine polyps. When the surgeon performed the operation, he found cancer throughout the abdominal area. He removed what he could and closed the abdomen. Miss C. lived with another single woman, Miss R., who was the same age but disabled from extreme obesity and other complications. Because Miss C. had no family, Miss R. represented her family and was able to discuss her fears about Miss C.'s illness with the social worker but not with the patient. Miss C. changed from being a healthy, working woman one day to being a terminally ill patient the next day. This was a catastrophic event for both parties, involving an overwhelming fear of abandonment for everyone. The patient denied the cancer and focused on the distress of the symptoms. Miss R. vented to the social worker. It was not easy to treat the patient (Miss C.) and family (Miss R.) as a unit of care. The worker understood that listening to Miss R. and paying attention to her somatic needs as well as the patient's concerns would be treating the patient and family together.

A study by Lack and Buckingham (1978, p. 95) supports the concept of patient and family as a unit of care. They found that family members who primarily carry the burden of care suffer more anxiety, depression, and social malfunctioning than the patients themselves. This was true in both hospice and nonhospice groups. Such objective data support the social work role in many health care settings, which is the importance of intervention with family members. In the previous case example, Miss R. was terrified of being left alone, and Miss C. was ignoring Miss R. and using denial to allow her to adjust to her radically changed living situation. In the interim, it was Miss R. who suffered the anxiety and depression and needed ongoing support from the social worker.

The ideal in hospice care is the patient and family as "patient." Hospice care operates on the assumption that there are intimate relationships, dependencies, and supports in the family relationships of the patient, and they affect care. Koff (1980, p. 33) states, "Hospice care recognizes that the way every member of the family deals with the dying of one of its community influences the way that person will die and the ability of the hospice to have impact on the death."

A social worker in a California hospice reports, "The more threads we can pull together for the patient and family, the easier the process becomes." The worker adds, "We help patient and family with financial, emotional, or physical problems. We help with unfinished business. We work on helping them be together." The worker concludes:

> We constantly redefine as a staff what is helpful and what is intrusive, and it's often very hard to know. The more we can remove the burden of isolation, pain, and loss of control, the easier the dying process can be. These things are all present for dying patients and families, and the less painful we can make each of those elements, the less stressful the dying will be.

Zimmerman (1981) supports these observations by stating that families of dying patients face problems that can seem overwhelming and can cause illness in family members. Some of these problems relate to the patient's illness; some problems are a result of the impending loss. Some are practical problems of finances and living arrangements. Others are psychological problems related to understanding and accepting altered life circumstances. Families need to be cared for by the team. Families begin at different levels of understanding and acceptance, and within each family there can be significant differences. Preconceptions on the part of family members, intrafamily hostilities, and uncertainty among health personnel regarding the nature of the patient's illness and prognosis can all serve as barriers to family members understanding the situation.

Since many hospices are home care services, the family takes on special significance. All the aforementioned concerns are present, but in the home setting the family is on familiar ground. The family member who is the primary caregiver for the terminally ill patient can help the hospice team, as well as receive help. Families usually know and understand the particular likes and idiosyncrasies of the patient. They may be open to help or resistant to it. Usually a terminally ill person is not accepted in a hospice unless a primary caretaker is in the home. The following, however, are two examples of hospice in varying settings in which social workers managed to circumvent this particular criterion.

The first example is a large urban hospital, from which the social worker reported that many patients were elderly and had no family. She was pleased to have been able to help some patients die at home by arranging a twenty-four-hour-a-day home health aide. The second example is an eastern suburban hospital in which a man was accepted into the hospice program before workers learned that he had no primary care person. The team decision was to keep him. The patient was a divorced man in his sixties whose children lived far away. He desperately wanted to go home to die. The social worker reported, "Everyone said we couldn't do it, but we managed it. He had some money, and he went home with private duty nurses, which he needed. We called on supports in the community—the church, neighbors, hospice volunteers. He died at home after ten days—pain free and where he wanted to be!"

Many times the patient is inaccessible to the worker. This can occur if the patient is comatose, heavily sedated, or enveloped in total denial. In such cases, the social worker contacts the family. The worker is aware of the risk the family is facing and will begin to engage the members in the process. Even if the worker develops a relationship with the patient, it is always essential to be in touch with the family. Bertman (1980, p. 341) states that dying is indeed a family affair but does not necessarily mean that the members comfortably support one another as they experience the process. Needs and concerns of the family members can be radically different from those of the person who is terminally ill. The patient may want to talk about how the family will manage when he or she dies, and the family may continue to talk about the future as if no one is dying. This, in fact, is the more common problem the worker has to face in most health settings. A patient can be days or hours from death, and the family is discussing the weather or is avoiding the patient.

A worker in a hospital gave an example. She was assigned to an elderly woman with a colostomy. The patient's husband had lost two previous wives, one to cancer and the other to heart disease. He sent his wife to the hospital to die because he and his stepdaughter could not cope with it. The worker visited the patient, who did not talk about dying but reviewed her life. It was unstated, but the worker and the patient knew that the worker had become the patient's surrogate family. The day she died, the worker tried to reach the husband and daughter but could not. Subsequently, she was able to comfort the husband and daughter in some small measure, but she perceived herself as being the family to this dying woman.

A seventy-year-old woman who was dying from breast cancer was admitted to the hospital. The social worker saw her several times, and she was in denial. On one particular day, when the social worker was reminiscing with Mrs. L., she began to cry; the worker silently held the patient in her arms. Mrs. L. said she was worried about what was going to happen to her husband when she was gone. The worker was beginning to explore this with Mrs. L. when her sisters arrived. They were so upset by their sister's tears that they went to the hospital administrator and told him not to allow their sister to be seen by any social worker. The patient was thereby deprived of visits by the one person with whom she could share her feelings; the social worker could not even explain her absence. This created an unresolved conflict for the social worker and a loss for the patient. When family members are frightened by emotional content, it forces the patient to comply with their needs, not her own.

Some family members are more available but need help in learning how and what to do in the face of losing someone they love. "We've been married for forty years. How will I manage without him?" "We had a fight the night before she went to the doctor. How can I make it up to her?" "We were just preparing to go away!" "How can she do this to me?" This is a sprinkling of some of the sentiments the social worker will hear. The social worker has to tune in to the expressed words as well as the unexpressed words. The family members may feel abandoned, angry, fearful, and uncertain. Time spent listening empathically to a family member who is emotionally upset or who has aches and pains can be productive for the patient, family, and worker.

Sometimes the social worker can connect the family members to the terminally ill patient. Family members who have been estranged can sometimes resolve bad feelings with the dying person because they learn to talk to one another in ways that were impossible until one member was dying. For example, Mrs. B. found that when her father was dying, they became close for the first time. He shared with her his own dreams for himself and for her and told her she had more than fulfilled them. Mrs. B. was initially overwhelmed but recovered and was able to tell her father how important and meaningful he had been during her life. After her father died, Mrs. B. was able to share with the social worker how healing it had been for her and her father to talk and share their feelings. She said, "If he had died without talking, I would have been left with nothing!"

If a patient is referred to a hospice, the first step for the social worker is to identify the family members who are involved with the patient and develop some understanding of their relationships with the patient and with one another. As family members are identified and relationships with the patient are clarified, it is time to ascertain if they understand the patient's illness and prognosis. Often this is a complicated process. Family members are at different levels of understanding and acceptance, as stated earlier, and sometimes put up barriers. Nonetheless, as the family members begin to understand the situation, their individual needs begin to emerge, and the hospice team can start to help meet those needs. As family understanding and acceptance grow, they become part of the team. Family members then can provide the patient with physical and emotional help. This is the goal and is very helpful to both the patient and the family. The social worker is often integral in helping achieve this goal.

As mentioned earlier, families can be intact, fragmented, blended, extended, or made up of unrelated individuals. Social workers are able to work with people in varying situations. A social worker in a California hospice gives an example that illustrates the complexities possible in any family group.

A woman in her fifties was referred for a home health evaluation. The nurse discovered when she went to the home that the husband was terminally ill also. They both had lung cancer. Theoretically, the wife's cancer was progressing much more rapidly, but it became clear that she was not going to allow herself to die before he did. She saw herself as being very much needed. They had a son who was drug dependent, and the social worker provided concrete services to obtain medical care, financial aid (Medicaid), attendant care, and oxygen. The worker also referred the son to psychiatric care. There was good close contact with the physician, and a niece with three small children was located as the nearest family. The husband died a few weeks after the hospice became involved with the family, and the social worker reported that the wife felt supported by the team. She was filled with tumors and continued to live with intractable pain. Finally she opened up and told the home health attendant that she was concerned about "sinning." The social worker brought a spiritual counselor to her, and after seeing the clergyperson, she was able to let go and died. The social worker reported everyone on the team was close to this woman, and they gave one another tremendous support to make her death bearable.

APPLYING THE HOSPICE CONCEPT IN THE HOSPITAL AND SKILLED NURSING FACILITY

It is hoped that hospice concepts can move into the hospital and skilled nursing facility. The hospital and skilled nursing facility can provide flexibility in visiting hours, in allowing people to bring personal items to their rooms, and in allowing family members to stay overnight with the dying person. Health teams can make efforts to include patient and family in care and treatment plans, which would ensure open communication. Pain control can be released from schedules, and concern for the health of family members can be attended to. Additionally, close ties should be developed between hospitals, skilled nursing facilities, home care, and hospices. In those facilities that include hospice units, learning takes place among health personnel.

A social worker in a large urban hospital that had a scatter-bed hospice (terminally ill patients in beds which the hospice team visited) within the hospital reports, "One of the most important things hospice is doing in this hospital is not related to any one patient or family but, rather, to care for patients in a general way. It is now permissible to deal with dying more openly, and people don't fall apart—neither staff, patient, nor 'family.'"

The attitudes of the social worker and others on the health team who care for the patient in hospitals and skilled nursing facilities play a vital role in determining whether denial will be used effectively. When the reality of the situation permits legitimate optimism for patient and family, hopefulness on the part of the social worker, nurse, or physician will help and encourage the patient to use denial. When optimism has no basis in fact, health personnel need to help the patient face reality rather than allow the patient to face the fearful experience alone. Rabin and Rabin (1985, p. 172) say optimism and hope must be founded on truth, but when truth dictates the inevitability of death, the patient must be helped to face the inevitable.

SUMMARY

It is necessary to keep in mind that the experience of life-threatening illness creates for the patient the need to cope with awesome demands just when biological and emotional resources are depleted by pain, fear, and loss of physical strength. For the family—depending upon whether the patient is a child, sibling, spouse, or parent— emotional resources, financial resources, and the energy for dealing with everyday management of family life may all be depleted by fear and the realities of the patient's condition (Germain, 1984, p. 63). If the social worker is able to listen and to hear the cues, the patient may or may not talk about his or her feelings as the need arises, and the family may or may not be able to talk without discomfort about the dying situation with the patient, the social worker, or the health staff. If the social worker is comfortable, then he or she can be helpful to dying patients and families even if they are not open. The social worker starts where the client is, whether it be denial, anger, or comfort. The social worker must accept the patient and family, work to understand the family complexities, and be available to the patient and family.

A discussion of working with the patient and family indicates the many aspects that must be considered. The many examples of practice in hospitals, skilled nursing facilities, and hospices operationalize those aspects. The worker needs to be aware of patients' needs and families' needs and, where possible, to work with patients and families as a unit of care. The process of dying can be experienced as meaningful for those involved; death does not have to be equated with failure. Those social workers who can bring their acceptance and availability to patients, families, and staff can bring to them the awareness that terminal illness is a part of the human experience.

Chapter 5

Grief:
Working with the Survivors

An understanding of grief is an integral part of working with terminally ill persons and their families. Grief is part of the dying person's life; grief is part of the family members' lives; grief surrounds all of them and envelops the survivors when the person dies. Each loss opens a void within each of us. The emptiness stretches ahead, and in the moment there seems to be no way to fill it.

DEFINING GRIEF

Grief and its attendant features have been discussed and listed by many scholars, researchers, and poets. The poets understood the phenomenon of grief long before mental health or health care professionals paid much attention to grief and the risks of that particular state. Hoagland (1984, p. 91) comments that since the loss of an important person universally elicits intense emotional responses, it almost seems that the job of describing the feelings associated with grief has been best left to poets and literature.

Systematic descriptions of bereavement from an objective and scientific point of view are difficult to achieve. It may be impossible to define a "typical" bereavement reaction, since so many variables contribute to the form and length of bereavement, as well as to the feelings of the bereaved. Also, bereavement behavior is defined in terms of social mores that vary greatly depending on culture, religion, and custom. What is considered normal in one society can be considered pathological in another. Bereavement is also defined by how tolerant the society is toward the grieving persons. Societal reaction can vary from "It's time to pull yourself together" after a few weeks to the enforced wearing of black (a sign of mourning) for the rest of one's life.

Historical Studies of Bereavement

A milestone marker of our society's concern for the bereaved occurred in the United States in the 1920s. Young widows were believed to be in need of financial assistance. This concern was the basis for the original Social Security legislation in the middle 1930s. Thomas Eliot (1930a, 1933), a social psychologist, wrote several articles on the bereaved family in the early 1930s and published a four-part, thirty-five-question interview to determine the experiences or observations of a bereaved family. Eliot (1930b, p. 115) pleaded for physicians, nurses, undertakers, ministers, and social workers to pool their knowledge and techniques for helping survivors work through bereavement. He also stated that issues of bereavement had been left to poets, artists, and composers, and he requested that social workers who read his article and were working with families write to him. Through these efforts, he attempted to systematize the grief experience.

Erich Lindeman (1944) was the major contemporary theorist to contribute to the understanding of survivor problems. He detailed some morbid grief reactions: (1) somatic distress, (2) preoccupation with the image of the deceased, (3) guilt, (4) hostile reactions, and (5) loss of normal pattern of conduct. He stated that when a person is willing to accept the grief process and to embark on a program of dealing, in memory, with the deceased person, a rapid release of tension can be achieved.

John Bowlby is another scholar who contributed to the understanding of loss, separation, grief, and bereavement. He developed some of his major theoretical work in 1960. Bowlby reviewed the literature and discussed separation anxiety in considerable depth from the psychoanalytic viewpoint, with particular attention to mother and child. He suggested that separation from mother has three phases: protest, despair, and detachment. Protest is the problem of separation anxiety, despair describes stages of grief and mourning, and detachment is a form of defense. In the case of grief in an adult, Bowlby regarded separation anxiety as a sign of the healthy personality.

Bowlby (1961, pp. 317-340) detailed the processes of mourning: (1) initial mourning, in which the individual experiences repeated disappointment, persistent separation anxiety, and grief; (2) disorganization of personality accompanied by pain and despair; and (3) reorganization, which is, in part, connection with the lost object and, in part, connection with a new object or objects. He further stated that although the sequences of behavior and feelings oscillate violently, there is a discernible trend from protest through despair to a new equilibrium of feeling and behavior. This whole subjective experience is grief. Grief, he stated, is a peculiar amalgam of anxiety, anger, and despair following the experience of what is feared to be irretrievable loss.

Hoagland (1984) points out that one of the most important discoveries about bereavement is that the symptoms tend to follow a predictable course over time. However, time is only a gross predictor because other variables, such as previous experience with loss, significance of the relationship with the deceased, and the extent of social supports available, interact to determine the reduction of symptoms.

Grieving has universal aspects that social workers and other counselors should understand. These phases of grief include shock and numbness; facing and accepting the reality of the loss, which includes yearning for the deceased; depression, and struggling with giving up emotional ties to the deceased; and reorganizing and developing new relationships. A primary grief lesson is understanding that attachment to the dead loved one goes hand in hand with letting go (Bernstein, 1997, p. 181). Also, each survivor has unique aspects. Each client's grief work will be unique to his or her personality and relationship to the deceased.

Mr. and Mrs. H. came to see a social worker six months after their twenty-six-year-old son, Roger, had died from Hodgkin's disease. The illness had been diagnosed six months prior to his death. Roger became ill when he was less than a year away from receiving his PhD in philosophy from Harvard University.

Mrs. H. reported to the social worker that she had nothing to look forward to, that there was nothing good at all in her life. She was losing her health and her ability to do things. She had lost her sex drive, her appetite, and her ability to concentrate since Roger died.

Mr. H. said he was very depressed and could stay in their house "forever" because it helped him remember Roger as he was— healthy and in his own surroundings. Mr. H. said, "Roger's death gave me a desire for death." Mr. H. was afraid of being alone, and he said he would need to "hunker down" to avoid those things which reminded him of Roger.

Both Mr. and Mrs. H. were professional people. He was an attorney, and she was a management specialist. They had a daughter who was in law school.

We can generally categorize grief as occurring in four stages: (1) shock and numbness, (2) yearning and pining, (3) depression and intense grief, and (4) reintegration. The social worker recognized from this first meeting with Mr. and Mrs. H. that they were experiencing the third stage of grief. Some of the manifestations of the intense grief stage include painful longing, preoccupation, memories, mental images of the deceased, a sense of the deceased being present, sadness, tearfulness, insomnia, anorexia, loss of interest, irritability, and restlessness (White and Gathman, 1973, p. 98). Grief may also uncover problems, in generally satisfactory lives, of which some people were unaware, and such problems may make it especially difficult to face the pain of grief resolution. For example, Mr. and Mrs. H. discovered that family was more important to them than their professional work lives, which caused considerable stress. Also, some secondary relationships, such as Mrs. H.'s relationship with her mother-in-law, although always poor, caused marital friction after Roger died.

THE RISKS TO SURVIVORS

Urban society tends to create alienation and to be nonaccepting of emotionality. Gorer (1965, pp. 150-151) notes that contemporary society wishes to ignore grief and treat mourning as morbid. He states that the work of mourning can be assisted or impeded, and its benign outcome facilitated or made more difficult, by the way the mourner is treated by society in general and, in particular, by friends and family members. He states that adults need help living through the phase of intense grief, but they rarely get it.

Studies demonstrate that bereaved persons are at much higher risk for physical and psychiatric illness than those who are not bereaved. Rees and Lutkins (1967, pp. 13-16) found a sevenfold increase in mortality risk between the bereaved and the control group, which was significant at the $P = .0001$ percent level. Of the bereaved group of close relatives, 4.76 percent died within one year of bereavement, compared with 0.68 percent in the control group. Parkes and Weiss (1983) report similar results for morbidity in bereaved individuals. Comparing the bereaved group with a married group, thirteen months after the loss of their spouses, the bereaved sample reported more physical disability and symptoms associated with the functioning of the autonomic nervous system. Such symptoms included trembling, nervousness, chest pain, sweating without cause, a persistent lump in the throat, dizziness or fainting, and palpitations. The identification of post-morbid expressions are clinically approachable and are credited for productive grief management (Powers and Wampold, 1994).

Many other studies have been built on those just described and support their data. Other studies explore effects of variables such as age of bereaved, length of illness of deceased, who died, place of death, and lifestyle. Parkes (1972), in his study of variables that might predict outcomes for American widows and widowers, concludes that intense grief, anger, and self-reproach present after six weeks may lead to diminished psychological, social, and physical adjustment a year later. In an earlier study, Parkes (1971) noted that widows in England reported gradual improvement in anxiety and depression over a three-year period. During the first year of bereavement, this cohort of thirty-eight widows spent more days sick in bed and had more admissions to hospitals than the nonbereaved. They showed more sleep and appetite disturbance, weight loss, and increased usage of alcohol, tobacco, and tranquilizers.

One of the major risks to survivors is experiencing the sudden or traumatic death of a family member or loved one. Any death that is not anticipated can fit this risk and may include suicide, homicide, random means such as accidental shooting, or car accidents. Multiple deaths can occur in car accidents, bombings (e.g., Oklahoma City and Kosovo), school shootings (e.g., Littleton, Colorado), famine, and natural disasters such as tornadoes, hurricanes, earthquakes, floods, etc. Unfortunately, such experiences are becoming more common.

Suicide has been a part of our society since its beginnings. In the early 1990s, there were an estimated 3.68 million surviving family members in the United States (McIntosh, 1993). Since a sense of shame is still attached to death by suicide, social workers and other counseling persons may need to be more proactive in reaching out to surviving family than is generally the case with other kinds of clients. Flexibility is an essential component for the social worker working with survivors. The social worker can provide support with reassurance and gentle affirmation of the reality of the death to the bereaved. Such persons can be referred to support groups for those bereaved by suicide. As in all loss, listening and being empathetic allows the survivor to give voice to the loss.

Many surviving family members of a loved one's suicide carry a special burden of grieving. They have higher levels of guilt, shame, and anger—only three of the emotions that such survivors can experience. The survivor is also left with questions such as why the loved one committed suicide and what, if anything, might have been done to prevent it. Such questions, usually unanswerable, may prolong the process of grieving and condemn surviving family to remain in the shadow of that death for longer than is healthy. Survivors also may struggle if they belong to a religious group that considers suicide a mortal sin. Such survivors need support from the community and may well need additional help with individual or group counseling (Stillion, 1996).

When the survivor is dealing with the homicide of a loved one, Redmond (1996) calls the reaction cognitive dissonance. The death does not make sense; the mind cannot comprehend or absorb its meaning. Other feelings are disbelief and murderous impulses, as well as conflict of values and belief systems. Survivors must cope with feelings of fear, vulnerability, anger, rage, shame, blame, guilt, and emotional withdrawal. In addition to all of this, the family must learn to deal with law enforcement, the criminal justice system, media intrusion, and defense attorneys. Grief likely will be prolonged and powerful. It may be some time before a survivor can begin to do grief work in a survivors group. The work in individual and group therapy is done to be able to come to terms with cognitive dissonance, murderous feelings, and sorting out the conflict of values and belief systems.

Sudden deaths are also caused by heart attacks and major strokes. Each year about 500,000 deaths are caused by some form of cardiac-related problem, and about 150,000 deaths result from strokes (Hersh, 1996). These numbers represent only a percentage of those who experience a heart attack or stroke, as some survive. Often such sudden deaths leave families in shock, and it takes longer to work through the grieving process. It is important for social workers to support such families over a period of time, perhaps for more than a year.

The problem of vehicular death, especially if caused by a drunk driver, is particularly severe. The minimal criminal sanctions that drunk drivers receive, as compared to those who kill with a gun or a knife, add to the difficulty of the families' grief, mourning, and recovery.

Vehicular crashes are another greatly unanticipated cause of death. A crash is a random event that has no reason and defies understanding. A further problem can be the form of notification, which can be by telephone. Not long ago, a young man was burned to death in a vehicular crash. "The law enforcement agency did not notify the family, and the man's father learned of his son's death when the medical examiner called him for dental records. The father was alone, and after hanging up the phone, he suffered a heart attack and died" (Lord, 1996, p. 27).

It is apparent that a social worker should always ask, "How did you find out about the death?" The survivor needs to repeat this experience of hearing the news over and over again. There was no chance to say good-bye and no opportunity for closure. Often survivors need to see the body, which may not be easy because police or medical examiners may make it difficult. The sense of helplessness from not knowing whether a loved one suffered is insurmountable (Lord, 1996). Over time, survivors may approach police about seeing pictures. Sometimes seeing pictures may be less horrendous than what the imagination had conjured up without them. People ask for pictures when they are ready; seeing photos of the deceased may help survivors get on with the grieving process.

Can one make a context of meaning for a senseless death? If one can, it is a significant component of recovery. A close friend's daughter was driving her grandchildren home from California to Salt Lake City, Utah. She had a car accident, and the oldest grandchild was killed. However, her bodily functions were maintained until they reached the hospital, and her parents opted to donate her organs. This can give meaning to a senseless death. Others find meaning in a personal faith journey—some through activism such as establishing a MADD (Mothers Against Drunk Driving) chapter or joining a local activism group, and some make lifestyle changes such as staying home more or saying "I love you" to other survivors. Creating a context of meaning out of the senseless does not erase the death or make it acceptable, but it does help survivors to appropriately honor and memorialize their loved one.

The social worker must help them live through the victimization by allowing the survivors to discuss it over and over again. The worker needs to accept all personal reactions and beliefs of the survivor. Whenever survivors feel ready, they should join a group of other people who have had the same experience. The social worker can be a supportive helper who is ready to help survivors as they make their journey toward a recovery that is never complete.

EXPERIENCING LOSS

Grief is universal. Understanding grief is connected to the cumulative loss theory as developed in Chapter 2. Each time a loss is experienced, the potential exists for a grief reaction. If one gives up a habit such as smoking, for instance, a loss is experienced. Part of the withdrawal symptoms of the smoker are reactions to the loss. Richard and Shepard (1981) reported that the biggest challenge for those who stop smoking is coping with feelings and emotions. They state that the loss of cigarettes is as acute as losing a friend. The feelings connected with the loss do not become evident until three to four months after cessation of smoking. They report that at that time, in their own experience of quitting, one of them felt a sense of sadness, although her personal and professional life was stable and pleasurable. Both felt a sense of acceptance of their losses about six to twelve months after smoking cessation. They had a conscious awareness of an end to a lifestyle that included smoking and a resolution of grief over a profound loss.

Giving up a substance such as tobacco, alcohol, caffeine, salt, etc., engenders feelings of loss and sadness. A physical loss, such as breast removal, leg amputation, hysterectomy, blindness, or deafness, will always engender grief. These losses are more common in hospital settings, and social workers who understand grief can help persons experiencing such losses.

The exact nature of bereavement and the amount of time involved remain unclear, although there is general agreement that loss of a significant loved one is usually associated with physical and psychological distress that can clearly reduce a survivor's functional status. There is no specific time in which bereavement can be resolved. It can last a few months to several years.

The bereavement experience is complex and involves the interaction of various factors, such as survivor response to loss, survivor characteristics, and external events. Social workers who can identify those factors, such as loss of income, pressure of dependent children, other losses, and job change, which have a measurable association with coping and which are clinically approachable are critical for productive grief management.

When children are bereaved, if they are included in the family plan, they feel acknowledged and supported by their families, which sets the stage for legitimizing their roles as mourners. Children can recognize the need for the ritual that acknowledges the worth of the deceased parent. The funeral helps greatly to acknowledge the death and serves as a place to share their feelings and to have those feelings accepted, and it is an opportunity to receive comfort from friends and family. The funeral is a place to say good-bye and perhaps feel close to the dead parent one last time, and a place for friends, family, and community to join the child or children in mourning. In participating in a funeral service that honors and memorializes the deceased, the process of internalizing a representation of the deceased has begun. This representation can change over time but begins with this experience (Silverman and

Worden, 1992). Grief resolution consists of complex tasks that place great demands on coping skills.

SOCIAL WORK ISSUES

Need to Review As Part of Healing

Mr. and Mrs. H. described to the social worker how they lived in a motel in Boston while their son, Roger, was in the hospital. When he was discharged, they hung curtains in his apartment, cleaned, and fixed up everything. After they returned to their home in Long Island, they went to Boston every other weekend. Roger seemed better, so they took a trip to Guadeloupe for a week. They received a phone call there that he had been rehospitalized, and they immediately returned to Boston. They stayed a month and went home a week before he was discharged from the hospital. He was rehospitalized again two weeks after discharge and died three weeks later. He experienced no pain or wasting away and died from a massive infection that resulted from the chemotherapy. Mrs. H. reported, "Roger said, 'It won't be bad for me if I die—it will be bad for you and Dad.'"

Mrs. H.'s ability to begin to review the circumstances shortly before Roger's death opened doors to the process of dealing with memories of the deceased. It is essential, in the early contacts with bereaved clients, to help them review the dying period in detail. This kind of review can be repeated over and over and is very helpful in moving beyond the immobility and despair created by the loss. Repetitive review of the details of the death is part of the process that helps the grieving person to work on the grief.

The Normal Process of Grieving

Existing confusion about what constitutes a typical grief reaction has been exacerbated by the increasing list of possible symptoms. Hoagland (1984, pp. 92-93) points out that Clayton and her colleagues found only three symptoms—depressed mood, sleep disturbances, and crying—that were acknowledged within a month after loss by more than half of their subjects. Hoagland further notes that the list of symptoms generated by Clayton and her colleagues is almost identical to the list of symptoms for a major depressive episode in the *Diagnostic and Statistical Manual of Mental Disorders* (DSM-III) of the American Psychiatric Association (1980).

Clayton, Desmarais, and Winokur (1974, p. 312) followed up their earlier study with one comparing mourning and depression. They conclude that, for research purposes, if the symptoms of depression occur only after the death of a loved one, the subjects should not be included in the group diagnosed as suffering from a primary affective disorder. Clayton, Desmarais, and Winokur (1968), in the earlier study, conclude that persons who sought psychiatric help for bereavement were different from the norm. Those who seek psychiatric care may be different, but I contend that all persons experiencing bereavement can use professional intervention, for one session or several sessions, if only to assure them that what they are experiencing is within the realm of normality. Facets of grieving, such as audio and visual hallucinations, are normal during the second stage of grief, but a person who does not know that may suffer severe stress.

Mr. H. told the social worker that he could hear Roger talking to him when he was in the library in his home. It was a frightening experience to him. The social worker told him that it was not unusual to hear the deceased person talking during the grieving period. He was greatly relieved. But what happens to people who see or hear their deceased loved ones and have no way of knowing it is normal or are afraid to talk to friends or family because they might be unwilling to listen?

Searching Behavior

A social worker in a university setting found out that a former student had lost her husband suddenly. He died from a heart attack at fifty years of age. The social worker sought out the student several weeks after the tragedy and spent a private hour with her. The student, Mrs. F., reported sadness, longing, fatigue, and apathy but was most upset when she had to go grocery shopping and found herself staring at all the men. The social worker explained to Mrs. F. that she was describing "seeking," which was very much within the normal expected behavior. She was looking for her dead husband. Parkes (1970) said that searching, by its very nature, implies the loss of an object; it is thought to be an essential component of grief and important to any understanding of the process. Mrs. F. was greatly relieved and weeks later reported to the social worker that after their talk she was able to cope with the loss more effectively. This example shows how just one session can help to move a grieving individual further along in grief work.

Grief Work

In the case of Mr. and Mrs. H., the social worker told Mr. H. at their third meeting that in six months he would have days without thinking of Roger and that he would not feel guilty. His memories would be positive, and although the death would always bring sadness, it would not bring pain. Mr. H. said he wanted to believe it and admitted that he was greatly relieved to learn that he was not crazy because he heard Roger's voice.

Mrs. H. wanted to repeat the discussion about Roger's illness. She said she wanted to move the clock back. Then she said, "I can't see Roger anymore!" Her experience was the opposite of that of her husband; she was losing the image of her son. She remembered that Roger had hope and had said to her, "If treatment is successful, I'll have two more good years." Mrs. H. said she sometimes felt over-whelmed by thinking about the anxiety Roger must have felt when he was sick. The social worker helped Mrs. H. to think about the warmth and nurturing she had provided during the time he was sick. Mrs. H. was able to review Roger's childhood years and to say she always had been frightened about his survival.

The foregoing is a description of the active process of grief work. Hodge (1971) comments that the word "mourning" is an active verb, and the duration of the process depends upon coming to grips with the pain and distress of grief work. The therapeutic principle is that the grief work must be done, that is, the basic depression must be addressed and worked through. If it is, growth can result; if it is not, illness may occur. Mr. and Mrs. H. were experiencing an un-complicated bereavement in DSM-IV terms, but it was greatly fa-cilitated by a professional counselor enabling them to confront the pain and fears engendered by the loss of their adult son. Such professional intervention can relieve anxiety and reduce the time necessary to work through the grief process.

Referral

It is presumed that the social worker has developed a relationship with the deceased prior to death and with the family or supportive persons who will be considered survivors. One of the pieces of data the social worker must have is whether the survivors have previously experienced the death of a loved one. Such data help the social worker to assess the resources survivors have to deal with the present death. If the setting, including some hospices, does not allow for ongoing bereavement counseling, it is very important to refer survivors to appropriate agencies or individual counselors who understand the needs of bereaved persons. Covill (1968) makes this suggestion for public health personnel and comments that such personnel can play a part in reducing the excess morbidity and mortality associated with bereavement by putting the bereaved in touch with a suitable agency.

Bereavement Services in the Institutional Setting

It is apparent that bereavement is a state of being that needs recognition and attention from health personnel. Hospice services usually have bereavement help for family members. A social worker or nurse coordinates the bereavement services, and the person who provides the service is often a trained volunteer. Hospices that cannot provide individualized bereavement counseling often offer group meetings or social events. The staff will frequently call family members on specific anniversaries that may create anxiety for the survivors.

In the more conventional setting, such as a hospital or skilled nursing facility, intervention at the time of bereavement may very well contribute to altering the subsequent outcome. Stubblefield (1977) describes such a prevention program in a Michigan hospital. She states that even when death has been long anticipated, the actual event is still often a shock to the family. After the family views the deceased, the social worker can discuss the grief reaction with the family and can describe some of the feelings family members can expect to experience over the next months. These experiences can include somatic distress characterized by sighing, weakness, feelings of unreality, distance from other people, and a tendency to be irritable; preoccupation with the dead person and feelings of guilt; and inability to concentrate, with disruption of normal routines. The family is also prepared for feelings of hostility toward the deceased, as well as the tendency of the bereaved to identify with various aspects of the deceased person.

Mr. S.'s wife died in the hospital from a brain tumor, and he was able to see the social worker on a weekly basis for ten weeks of bereavement counseling. The social worker had helped Mr. S., before his wife died, with the grief problems he could expect after her death and with the problems their four children would encounter. Since Mrs. S. was comatose for the last five weeks of her life, much of the grief work with Mr. S. and the children could begin in anticipation of her death. The social worker knew that when a spouse or other family member dies, the loss is experienced as a threat to one's very identity; it is as if a part of the self vanishes with the deceased (Uroda, 1977).

Unfortunately, social workers providing help to the bereaved are not the norm in hospital practice. The patient dies, and the case is closed. Thus, the informed and caring social worker may want to invest time and effort in changing policy decisions to allow for intervention with survivors after the patient has died. In skilled nursing facilities, social workers should be working with residents who were close to the bereaved patient. Most hospice programs have a bereavement protocol. For example, Hospice of Pennsylvania, Inc., works with bereaved families through one-to-one visitation, phone calls, written correspondence, workshops, and memorial services (McDonnell, 1986, p. 261). Social workers are uniquely qualified to administer bereavement counseling programs in hospices. Formal and informal supportive and therapeutic services should be part of every hospice and follow survivors for twelve to eighteen months after the death of the patient. McDonnell (1986, p. 226) states that the whole population benefits from humanistic health care practices.

Issues of Timing

It is crucial for social workers in health settings such as hospitals or skilled nursing facilities to understand the needs of survivors and the ways in which such persons can be helped to move into the necessary grief work. Grieving is accomplished by the psyche, either immediately, over a reasonable period of time, or over a much extended period of time. The sooner the grief work is begun, the more quickly the survivors can reorganize their lives and move on to new and different lives. When grief is extended, repressed, or manifested in bizarre behavior, it is often classified as pathological grief (which is discussed later in this chapter). The point is that social workers must be aware of the time factors and must make every effort to engage survivors either before or at the moment of death.

Another issue of timing relates to people's ability to receive help. From our knowledge of grief stages, we already know that the initial stage is often shock and denial. People who experience such reactions do not respond to immediate help. Societal norms of funeral, wake, shivah, and mourning periods tend to wrap around survivors so that a week or ten days after death, when the shock is lessened and the survivor is alone, the second stage descends, often with catastrophic effects on the bereaved. Krant (1973, p. 289) makes an eloquent plea for a hospital unit of social workers, clergypersons, psychologists, and psychiatrists to work in tandem with the medical physician during the dying process and after death. He states, "It may require considerable conviction and ingenuity either to have 'grief' classified as a disease, or to alter payment systems to acknowledge prevention-intervention as legitimate." If grief is conceptualized as a normal part of the bereavement process, then funding of bereavement services is a necessary corollary to providing services to terminally ill persons and their families.

Different issues of timing are related to a couple of the major killers of the twentieth century. Adults who survived the devastation of the Nazi Holocaust or the annihilation of Hiroshima and Nagasaki had the experience of living through indescribable horrors. Survivors had no way to understand what had happened to them because the events were beyond our language's ability to describe, much less explain to these survivors. These were adults faced with realities for which they had no words, no concepts, and no stories, adults who felt helpless to make sense of the catastrophes that had changed their lives forever (Harris, 1995). The Hebrew word "Shoah," another name for the Holocaust, means catastrophe. A catastrophe is a great and sudden calamity, a complete failure, a sudden, violent change in one's life.

It took fifty years to begin discussing and to start releasing some of the feelings of the survivors of the Holocaust and the atomic bombings.

The death of a parent can be just as agonizing to a young child. It is the most devastating of the off-time events (a person who dies before becoming old) of grief any person experiences. Children are "at a loss for words." Even if children have the necessary vocabulary to talk about their loss, the flood of feelings, described by one adult as a tidal wave, is strong enough to overcome any conceptual abilities that do exist. Most important, similar to adult survivors of the Holocaust and the atomic bombings, the children have no story, no organizing text, with which to process their loss (Harris, 1995). The adult survivors of a parent's early death know the event by its enormity. Nothing in the child's life remained untouched. It was an absolute catastrophe. If a loved and needed parent can go away forever, is anything safe, predictable, or certain anymore? The loss permeates the inside and engulfs the person completely.

Most people who have suffered an early parental loss remember the day their world changed forever. Personal time is marked in terms of "before" and "after." This divide continues throughout life. Thirty, forty, or fifty years after the death, men and women still refer to the early death of a parent as the defining event of their lives. The language that adults use to describe the experience of losing a parent in childhood is the language of catastrophe, devastation, and emptiness.

Social workers need to explore with adults their experience with death and whether they were children when a parent died; the social worker knows what a devastating loss it was. The feelings may be reawakened by another terminal illness or death in the family. In fact, those who do not understand the previous loss and how powerful its effect was for the individual may wonder at that individual's extreme reaction to a subsequent death. It is important for social workers to know the unique circumstances of the situation.

Customs about death, funerals, and grief are universal to a degree. In all cultures, Western and Eastern, rituals are very necessary in attenuating the severity of grief reactions. Individuals in societies that perform final ceremonies some time after a person's death experience less severe grief, and those in societies that lack final postburial ceremonies have more prolonged grief (Parry, 1995).

Economic Issues

The National Hospice Organization struggled for years to have Medicare reimbursement extended to cover hospice services. In the early 1980s a bill was passed in Congress, but no reimbursement was included for bereavement counseling. In the summer of 1983, Congress set the limit for Medicare payments for hospice patients at $6,500. There has been an ongoing struggle since 1983 to keep the rates from being eroded in a climate of constant cost cutting. Since grief is not classified as a disease, the option was to alter payment systems to acknowledge prevention and intervention for bereavement. The payment systems have been altered, even with an acknowledgment of the need for counseling, and a few programs provide bereavement services as part of a funded hospice program. However, in a time of resource limitations, the funding of preventive services tends to get lost.

PREVENTION

Bereavement services can be thought of as prevention. If bereavement services are able to help people cope more effectively with the possible physical and emotional morbidity associated with survivorship, then such services qualify as prevention.

The concept of prevention is strongly supported in pediatric units, in which the death of a child can cause major emotional, physical, and social dislocation for parents and siblings (McCollum and Schwartz, 1972). The process of grief for parents who lose a child can go on for years. Intervention during the dying process and soon after death can be very helpful. Prevention must also be considered for the caring health team members, since the multidisciplinary staff members experience grief, and survivor conferences can help them (Whitt et al., 1981-1982). The important concept is the ongoing intervention provided for the dying person and for those persons who are deeply involved on an emotional level with the dying person, both family and staff. The importance of finding meaning in life may have a concurrent relationship with change occurring in the greening process (Edmonds and Hooker, 1994). The social worker provides the ongoing process of counseling, concrete help, being available, and preparation for grief during the lifetime of the dying person. If the social worker cannot provide ongoing counseling for family members after the person's death, then availability by telephone or referral to grief specialists can be provided.

A body of research was completed with a series of studies at the University of California at San Francisco Medical School. The group studied was composed of patients who came for therapy six months after the death of a parent. They were compared with a group of people whose parents had died and who had not sought therapy. Over the course of the year, the symptoms of distress among those in therapy declined to the level of those in the comparison group. The major change that seemed to have brought about their improvement was being able to actively confront the feelings and thoughts their parents' death evoked, that is, to mourn (Goleman, 1985). These studies support the notion that counseling is a preventative for the bereaved, who are at risk for excessive rates of morbidity and mortality.

Benoliel (1971) comments that it is not enough for members of the health care team to recognize the signs of grieving and respond in ways that facilitate the process; they must also be available to individuals at times when they are ready to use this kind of help, which is usually after the survivors no longer are in contact with the hospital; "yet the health care system as it is now organized provides little in the way of systematic transition care for many individuals adapting to a personal loss that is catastrophic in its effects" (p. 190). The ability to offer help on the spot, although it may not be accepted at the time, may encourage a person to seek help when needed. It is also important to offer to be available at a later time when the person may need a social worker. Rabin and Pate (1985) state that families who have experienced a death in the hospital should be informed about other resources available in the community to help them cope with their emotional crisis. Also, the family should be told explicitly that they can return to the emergency room for follow-up care if necessary. Hospital social workers give information and referral services and can provide bereavement services to survivors, but only if they return to the hospital.

COUNSELING SURVIVORS

Mr. and Mrs. H., who had been told about specialists in grief counseling by the hospital social worker when their son died sought out a professional who could help with bereavement. On the fifth visit, Mr. and Mrs. H. both told the social worker there had been a real change for the better. This quick change may be related to their readiness to accept help.

Mrs. H. reported thinking less about Roger's death and being able to let her mind go elsewhere. However, she said she felt more uptight. Her frustration tolerance was very poor, and her compulsiveness had increased. She wanted to get things done and over with and felt she had no time to relax and enjoy anything. The social worker asked how this manifested itself. Mrs. H. said she talked too much and needed to fill all the gaps. Roger's death had caused a breakdown in self-esteem; her person was diminished, her ego deflated. Her major values of family and parenting were extremely shaken up. She asked herself, "What is it all about?" She felt less secure in everyday situations. She remarked that this was a "tough" time of life (even if Roger were alive); i.e., the children were gone, aging was beginning; she wanted grandchildren and that possibility had been cut in half.

Mr. H. said things were better for him, and he didn't know if it was time, the social worker's help, or something else, but life was much better. He was slowing down and not feeling he had to go at such a frenetic pace. He commented that Roger's death had caused him to become more interested in his own affairs and that he was not afraid of his own death. He said, "Having a son at Harvard and a daughter at Princeton is pretty good for a guy who did CCNY [City College of New York] at night!" Mr. H. said his daughter was doing very well and was beginning to bloom as a professional and as a person. "She really enjoys law," he said. Mr. H. was getting great pleasure from her but was afraid it would be taken away. Mr. H. was more compassionate toward people he knew who had illnesses. He had less tolerance for trivial talk and was more appreciative of human values. He commented that Mrs. H. always perceived herself as the perfect mother, and he expected her to fall apart when Roger died; he was amazed at her strength. He ended the conversation by saying he felt he needed to get the best out of life.

The middle phase of grief work and therapeutic intervention shows the vacillation of the mother and the more reorganized response of the father to the loss of their adult son. They reviewed the death several times and expressed feelings of anger, guilt, constriction, and meaninglessness. They were able to verbalize feelings and receive validation from the social worker that their feelings were normal and an expected part of grief work. Hauser and Feinberg (1976) suggest that during the middle phase of grief, the threat to one's own self becomes a reality, with the recognition of the loss of emotional and interpersonal ties previously invested in the lost one. The bereaved may now express thoughts of losing sanity and of life that no longer seems meaningful. The counselor helps by stating that what is being experienced is a reaction to be expected at this time.

Bereavement groups are much more common than individual help, particularly groups for widows and widowers. Bereavement groups are conducted by many hospice programs, and many of them are self-help groups. The nonwidowed social worker has a very legitimate role in such groups. Social work leadership carries the knowledge of grief and mourning, the understanding of the group process, and the concept of membership. Nonwidowed leadership brings objectivity and individualizes the expression of feelings among members (Anger, 1981, p. 311).

Mrs. D., whose forty-five-year-old husband died of a brain tumor, had attended a widow's group at her local library a few weeks after her husband's death. She came for individual help more than two years later because she had so many ambivalent feelings toward her husband and could not share those feelings in the group. The group, however, helped her to take over the household responsibilities, provided ideas to help her cope with her two sons, and encouraged her to meet other men. It was the breakup of a relationship with a man that brought her to individual counseling to complete the transition of her grief work.

Western society has a clear ethos about terminal illness. Death is perceived as a terrible event for an individual, and much energy is put into denying reality, even when the person is seriously ill. The terminally ill person must struggle with the emotional pain of grieving and the emotional distress of coming to terms with the prospect of having to die (Parry, 1990). The onset of an illness or a terminal diagnosis is a stark and sudden reminder of the finite nature of all human life. It triggers a reexamination of who we are, why we are here, and what we are doing. It forces us to confront questions of the limited time we have and how we are using that time. It forces us to look at relationships, including spiritual ones.

Doris Howell, an MD who is an oncologist, said, "The end-of-life choice is one most of us aren't prepared to make. There's so much silence to dying. We are not literate in planning or saying good-bye" (Morgan, 1999, p. A3). Dr. Howell joined the board of the San Diego Hospice twenty-five years ago and feels hospice offers people the promise that they do not have to die alone or in pain. It is believed that American mores focus excessively on extending doomed lives. The University of California at San Diego (UCSD) is in the first wave of medical schools requiring training in the care of the dying. Every third-year student at UCSD receives instruction at San Diego Hospice (Morgan, 1999).

The use of group work, family work, couples intervention, and individual counseling are all part of the techniques and practice the social worker brings to work with terminally ill persons and their family members. However, social workers need the support of the institutions in which they work.

It pays to educate the institutional hierarchy, which includes administrators and attending physicians, about the benefit of groups. This may take time, as discovered by Parry and Kahn (1976) when starting a group for emphysema patients in a community hospital. When group members report to their doctors or write letters to the hospital administrator about the benefit of groups, then the support for groups will increase. However, if physicians have a negative attitude toward groups, expressing concerns that members will get incorrect medical information or will become overanxious, it is very difficult to proceed with groups. A helpful way social workers can approach the problem is to put the plan for the group on paper and circulate it to the concerned physicians and administrators and ask for input from them.

PATHOLOGICAL GRIEF

Both Engel (1961) and Krant (1973) raised the question, "Is grief a disease?" Uncomplicated grief is a period of distress and discomfort and should receive the attention of both health care providers and close friends and family. However, pathological grief can be diagnosed with responses such as absence of grief, delayed grief, unresolved grief, ongoing depression, psychotic or neurotic reactions, pain, conversion symptoms, and other organic disease.

Hoagland (1984) points out that the DSM-III system clearly suggests that "complicated" bereavement (i.e., pathological grief) does not exist and is, in fact, something else, such as a major depression or a somatoform disorder. One could make a case for labeling pathological grief as a psychiatric disorder that is brought about by grief but has moved beyond the grief. However, this does not take into account the various states mentioned earlier, because the absence of grief or delayed grief would not easily fit into a psychiatric category. It may also be splitting hairs to decide whether the excessive grief reaction that becomes a psychiatric disorder would have occurred if the death that caused the grief reaction had not occurred.

Parkes, a psychiatrist, has written extensively on pathological grief in the English-speaking world. Parkes (1975) notes that the most common form of psychiatric illness is "chronic grief," and it is very severe. He states further that the criteria for predicting poor outcome in grief situations include low socioeconomic status and multiple life crises (particularly if they involve disturbance of the marital relationship) in the bereaved's life. Another factor that may precipitate chronic grief is if the person who died succumbed after a short-term illness with little warning of impending death.

I know of cases in which survivors kept a room, an entire apartment, or a house exactly as it was the day the person died. Such persons are fixated and frequently need psychiatric hospitalization. Behavior may be bizarre and can include outlandish dress and delusions, e.g., wearing all the clothing of the deceased or leaving everything of the deceased in place until he or she returns. This can be a brief reactive psychosis or a schizoaffective disorder.

Some people do not grieve and become wrapped up in the stoic image. There is also general agreement that ambivalent relationships often lead to severe grief reactions (Vachon, 1976). After twenty years of marriage, Mrs. D.'s husband died of a brain tumor. Mrs. D. went to a social worker three years after his death because she had ended a relationship with another man. She first began to review her husband's death, which she had delayed for three years. Mrs. D. needed to work through her feelings of loss, both negative and positive. Her husband's illness was difficult, and she was relieved when he died. Her ambivalence caused her to delay her grieving until a second loss occurred.

Social workers can help clients who experience pathological grief reactions if they realize that this is what the clients are presenting. Often the client presents with other complaints, and the social worker needs to be alert to losses in the past that may be unresolved or delayed. Barry (1973) states that the therapy of prolonged grief reactions consists of uncovering and abstracting the grief that has been held in abeyance.

The description of neurotic grief in the literature differs from that given here, in that there is no question in the examples cited here that clients are experiencing grief over a serious loss. Neurotic grief is excessive and disproportionate in nature. Usually the survivors recognize their reactions are excessive and unyielding, and the reaction itself then becomes a source of stress. Also, it is accompanied by irrational despair and feelings of persistent hopelessness. Such individuals feel the deceased died on purpose as a rejection of them. Further, they feel the death is their fault. Neurotic grievers have a limited ability to transfer their needs to others and remain stuck, with prolonged apathy, irritability, or aimless hyperactivity (Wahl, 1970). These kinds of survivors are not easy to assist. They need to be helped to understand their dependency on the deceased and the ways in which to free themselves for autonomous living. This involves longer-term therapy than helping survivors with uncomplicated bereavement.

The social worker held a terminating interview with Mr. and Mrs. H. two months after their initial meeting. Mr. H. said he had been helped tremendously. He went on to say that his hate was mostly gone, his sadness was reduced, and his anger was minimal. Mrs. H. said she felt similarly. She could wake up in the morning and not always think of Roger. The social worker discussed the unveiling ceremony that was to occur in a few weeks (a Jewish ceremony occurring one year after death). Mr. and Mrs. H. were able to resolve their differences about whether it should be private or open. The social worker explained that the process she had gone through with them over the two-month period was one of open communication.

Mr. and Mrs. H. had found that many of the familiar and taken-for-granted signposts and starting points of their daily lives no longer existed. They still needed time and help and were still struggling to rebuild and to grasp the full scope of this disruption to their lives. They were told during the therapy that the bad times would be the anniversary of Roger's death, his birthday, and holidays they had shared together. The simple discussion of the tendency of grief to recur on such occasions can be far more helpful than medications to alleviate specific symptoms.

SUMMARY

The discussion of working with survivors is complicated but indicates specific phases of grief that provide the practitioner with guidelines for helping. Grief has many facets, but an understanding of the process helps the social worker to meet the individual needs of the survivor.

Social workers understand the concept of family equilibrium and can assist survivors to learn how to rebalance their family equilibrium. This is a most important way of providing compassionate care to people who are experiencing emotional confusion, pain, and emptiness.

Chapter 6

Transitions and Reflections

A social worker in a hospice in California responded in the following manner to a question about how it feels to work with dying patients:

> It goes in cycles—the stress is high. I cope with it by being there physically, giving information, going through the motions, and withdrawing emotionally. Inevitably, there is one patient who breaks through and gets to me emotionally. There have to be rewards or I couldn't manage. Actually, working with dying patients gives me the most profound rewards of any in medical social work. Why? Because games drop by the wayside, rapport comes easily and is so meaningful. I see real changes in families.

Working with the terminally ill can be both stressful and rewarding. If a worker helps a dying patient to talk openly with close family members and friends, it is rewarding for patient, family, and social worker. If the social worker can help survivors grieve and move on to rebuild their lives, it provides mutual satisfaction for clients and worker. Throughout the foregoing chapters, it has become apparent that working with the terminally ill and their families is a complicated process. It is a process that requires a full understanding of the concept of cumulative loss and an awareness that denial can mean health.

TRANSITIONS

The concept of transition is most useful for social workers, patients, and families. Transition can be considered as the positive side of loss. One can lose childhood as one moves into adolescence, or one can experience the transition from childhood to adolescence. Transition presents the idea of moving from one place to another— from school to college, college to job and marriage, adulthood to parenthood, life to death. Also, within each loss there is a gain; one gains adulthood from adolescence, for example.

Parkes (1971) states that losses and gains are two ways of classi-fying changes in state. The implication is that loss is negative—that it leaves one in a worse state—whereas gain is positive, and one achieves a better state of being. Parkes goes on to say that the state depends upon the evolution of the outcome, and in certain major changes, the pros and cons balance out so that neither loss nor gain predominates.

If one perceives change as the mover that creates losses and gains, losses can provide relief and gains can suggest hazards. When a woman gives birth to her first child, she loses her life without children and she gains the state of parenthood. It can be a relief to lose the childless status; on the other hand, for many women, the birth of a child (gain) can create major stress. Parkes (1971) states that whether the situation is seen as a gain or loss, one is tempted to think that the crucial factor may be the way in which the individual copes with the process of change.

As we use this concept of transition—changes from one state to another—to examine the world of terminally ill persons, we can see that transition may encompass a change of catastrophic proportions. Dying patients need to marshal their resources to cope with the altered state. If the changes from being sick to being terminally ill take place gradually and individuals have time to prepare, little by little, for the rearrangement, the chances that transitional moves will follow a satisfactory course are greater than they would be if the changes are sudden and unexpected.

Mr. F. and Mrs. K., who were discussed in Chapter 2, are exam-ples of the difference between a gradual versus sudden change to terminal illness. Mr. F. had a two-year terminal illness and was involved in counseling for most of that time. Mr. F., his wife, and his adult children all had time to process the altered conditions that the illness brought into their lives. Mrs. K., on the other hand, received the diagnosis of cancer four months before she died and was assaulted with pain and the terrible symptoms of vomiting and constipation. Mrs. K. never really had time to process the tremendous loss she had to face. Her children, who were available, saw little of her, and when she died it was a profound shock to them. Half of her adult children were scattered around the country and were not able to provide her with much support during the terminal phase of her illness. Her sister was present, and the social worker was very available. Mr. F. vacillated between depression on his "down" days and feeling good when he was able to do more. Mrs. K. experienced severe physical symptoms but fought steadily against the illness.

Mr. F. made the transition from an active husband, father, grandfather, and artist to a passive participant in the familiar roles. However, he resisted leaving the artist role. He painted a large canvas, approximately seven by four feet, of his deceased parents before he gave up oils to settle for watercolors and inks. The transition from active to passive family member was made gradually, and eventually he developed much stronger and more vital relationships with his wife and children. He experienced severe emotional pain as his ability to practice his art was reduced.

Mrs. K. made an abrupt transition from active parent, active head of household, and breadwinner to frightened, angry, dependent patient. Four dependent children (ages fourteen, fifteen, sixteen, and seventeen) were living at home, and one son in his twenties took over running the household. Mrs. K. had so many responsibilities—her children, her sister, her mother—that death represented the last major battle she would have to fight. The transition was abrupt and overwhelming.

In the transitional sense, Mr. F. had many changes, ups and downs, twists and turns, and was moving forward and backward as he experienced the period of living with dying. Mrs. K. experienced similar ups and downs, twists and turns, but they were much more condensed. Germain (1984, p. 183) comments that the experience of living with dying must be viewed as a life transition. Additionally, terminal illness presents biological changes, physical pain, emotional pain and fears, grief, possible changes in the physical setting, sometimes emotional withdrawal of staff and/or family, and difficult medical procedures.

One of the most critical components of the life transition of dying is time. The time can be years, as with Mr. F.; months, as with Mrs. K.; or weeks, hours, or instantaneously, as in a fatal crash, suicide, homicide, or massive heart attack. One is reminded of Pattison's (1977) death trajectories (see Chapter 2) and the fact that the greater the uncertainty, the greater the stress for the family and patient. However, it is generally the case that if the terminal patient has more time, the transition is slower, and the family and patient have a better chance to process and come to terms with the many changes in their lives.

Transitions in the Hospice Setting

The hospice is often put forward as the answer to the dilemmas facing health care professionals in hospital settings. However, the ability of hospice to help dying patients make that transition from active living to reduced active living depends on the individual's ability to use that help. Hospice has many enthusiastic supporters who tend to view it as the panacea for all terminally ill patients. Unfortunately, this is not the case. Some terminally ill patients refuse hospice care because they are in total denial, and any attempt to break into that denial may be contraindicated. Most hospices require that patients being admitted know and understand their diagnosis and prognosis. If a person is referred to hospice and is in complete denial, the services would not be helpful. Also, some patients have physicians who will not refer them to hospice. This can result from a "wait and see" attitude about new problems, a feeling that their patients are already receiving holistic care, and a feeling that referring a patient to hospice will take away the patient's hope (Corr and Corr, 1983, pp. 340-341).

Some patients do not live close enough to a hospice to make use of it. There are also unresolved conflictual issues between the traditional medical system and the hospice. The physician in an acute care hospital who feels that aggressive medical care is required until death is in sharp contrast to the hospice physician, who is concerned with pain and symptom control within a quality-of-life approach. Also, involving the patient and family as a unit of care is a radical notion to many primary care physicians. The hospital is geared to cure and short-term stays; the hospice is geared to palliation and long-term care, if necessary.

A look at the facilities that provide care for terminally ill patients reveals the move from home to the institutional setting and back to the home with the hospice team. Within each institutional setting, new problems have affected the way terminally ill persons are treated.

Because of advances in medical technology, what was once a straightforward path to death is now a complex maze. Doctors now wonder when and whether to disconnect respirators, to resuscitate, to start special feedings, to treat infections, to withhold dialysis, or to continue transfusions. In some cases, doctors have called the hospital's lawyers to help determine when and how patients should die (Kleinman, 1985).

McDonnell (1986, p. 202) asserts that the hospice movement brings many challenges to health care practitioners and administrators. Hospice representatives in both systems advocate high-quality care that stresses palliation over technology for the terminal patient. The hospice orientation is humanistic in its concern for the well-being of the patient and family. Zimmerman (1981, p. 10) comments that hospices focus upon life and living rather than on death and dying: "They view death as a natural part of life, but as one which, like birth, can be made easier by the provision of some help."

Transitions for the Survivor

Death is one of the transitions of life. Once the dying person has completed the transition to death, the survivors begin their own transition into grief. As mentioned earlier, their transition can be a very abrupt and devastating experience. A patient is frequently brought to the emergency room in a hospital with trauma or a heart attack. If the emergency room has a social worker, the social worker is usually the professional person who spends time with the family while the medical staff is involved with providing lifesaving medical procedures that may or may not help. It is the social worker's job to develop a relationship over the hours of waiting and then to accept whatever behavior is exhibited by family members if the patient dies.

If the transition from death to grief occurs in this fashion, the period of shock and numbness may be more extended than for family who have had some anticipatory grieving time. Nevertheless, the family experiences the transition from fear to grief. This transition takes place by moving through almost total denial to a phase of bitter pining and frustrated searching for the lost person, assuming it is a normal grief reaction. This is followed by depression and apathy when the bereaved accepts the loss as a reality, and then a final phase of reorganization when new plans about the world and the self are made.

The previous chapter detailed this grieving transition for Mr. and Mrs. H. They were into the transition when they came for help. Mr. H.'s main concern was his auditory hallucinations. As Vachon (1976, p. 40) points out, in a study of 294 bereaved people, 47 percent stated the hallucinations were helpful. Thus, when Mr. H.'s feared hallucinations were explained as normal, the hallucinations ceased and then ultimately helped in his transition from bereavement to reorganization. Mrs. H. was experiencing the depression and apathy stage when she came for help. As she repeatedly reviewed the circumstances of her son's death, she was able to make the transition from bereavement to reorganization.

Persons experiencing transitions are particularly vulnerable. As a social worker in a hospital, I once heard a terrible keening coming from the emergency room. I hurried to the area and found the nurses wringing their hands and two women keening loudly. I found out their husband and father had just died from a massive heart attack. It seemed to me that the nurses needed more attention than the family members who were giving vent to their feelings. They were reacting to the abrupt wrenching from their lives of a loving husband and father who was suddenly dead. The transition from shock to grief would come soon enough.

As the social worker who was available to the keening family, I could only offer help when they felt ready to ask for it. I confirmed the normality of their reaction and helped the nurses realize that it would end soon and that we should not interfere with their spontaneous outburst, which was their way to relieve unbearable pain. The transition from acute pain of abrupt loss to the more pervasive pain of grief would come soon enough. What is required of the social worker in this situation is successful management of the critical challenge. The social worker in these emergency situations approaches these painful areas carefully and is available for the crises that may arise as persons move from one transition to another.

The challenge is the crisis created by sudden death. The shock to the family equilibrium is pervasive. It is referred to as dismemberment (Hill, 1967), and the family in crisis becomes susceptible to the influence of others in the environment (Rapoport, 1966). Thus, it is important for social workers to be available when the crisis is created by sudden death, when families are more susceptible to intervention. Successful management of the challenge requires providing support and caring, which enables individuals to mobilize energy for reacting to others in their family support network. Social work support in emergency room situations approaches family members carefully to determine what they can take in, who is able to take charge, and to assess the overall situation.

The emergency or trauma unit may have a standard operation mode in which social work service is available to family members in crisis, and if not, the social work department can work out their availability with emergency room staff. This can be an on-call routine for evening and weekend coverage. In the example of the keening family, the social work department was adjacent to the emergency area, and I heard the keening and hurried there to see if I could help. Thus, it was fortuitous that the social work department was placed in that location and that it was a weekday during working hours. There was an on-call arrangement, but social work would not have been called for a keening family. The family would have been hurried out of the hospital, and their transition from the abrupt loss of their husband and father to grief would have been even more painful.

EUTHANASIA, PHYSICIAN-ASSISTED DYING, LIVING WILLS, AND PATIENTS' RIGHTS

An inevitable question comes up when discussing hospice, which is the question of euthanasia. It is often defined as an easy and painless death when one is suffering from a terminal illness, thus causing some to equate it with hospice, which is living in a comfortable, pain-free manner. Euthanasia is not usually considered an option by patients or staff because the commitment in hospice is to living while dying.

Euthanasia is often considered an option by individuals in their own homes or by individuals and families in acute care hospitals. In one's own home, euthanasia becomes synonymous with suicide. In the acute care hospital, discontinuance of life-sustaining measures, such as respirators and intravenous feeding, is part of the discussion of euthanasia and physician-assisted dying. It is the fact of medical technology that has made euthanasia a commonly discussed issue. In 1999, Oregon voted on and passed an initiative to allow physicians-assisted suicide with the agreement of the patient.

Euthanasia is sometimes described as active or passive. Russell (1977) also describes a voluntary versus an involuntary euthanasia and says this is an incomplete and objectionable classification. At the heart of the debate is the concern that terminally ill persons should not be subjected to excessive technological prolongation of life, particularly if the person has made a specific request not to be kept alive by whatever medical technology is available. The concern for hospice patients is similar but is focused on providing relief from chronically distressing symptoms.

Russell (1977, p. 34) notes that, under present law, doctors are more and more often faced with the dilemma of having to choose between allowing prolonged suffering or mercifully granting a request for death in violation of criminal law. She goes on to warn that to think death will be easy and dignified if only doctors refrain from prolonging life by heroic efforts is a delusion. People will continue to suffer, in great distress and indignity, unless active steps are taken to induce death. The discussion has changed very little in twenty-three years. Even now the Oregon initiative is being challenged.

Each state has a Natural Death Act. The law addresses terminal illness, severe injury, and administering or withholding life support (Hoffman, 1994). The living will has come to be called an advance directive and is closely tied to the concept of euthanasia. The advance directive has been promoted by various groups, but the Euthanasia Education Council was responsible for its inception and drafting (Russell, 1977, p. 18). When my husband was admitted to a hospital in February 2000 he was asked if he had an advance directive for health care. The advance directive can provide physicians with some idea of the patient's intent and can help to relieve families of some of the burden of decision making. A person's wishes can be deduced from an advance directive, religious belief, or a consistent pattern of conduct, and life-sustaining treatment may be withdrawn if "there is some trustworthy evidence that the patient would have refused treatment and . . . it is clear that the burdens of the patient's continued life with the treatment outweigh the benefits of that life for him" (Annas, 1985). This is what the Natural Death Act is about.

A document that is legally binding is a durable power of attorney for health care decisions, which establishes a surrogate decision maker. The person with the decision-making ability can be a court-appointed guardian, a spouse, adult children, or adult siblings. If a patient has no family members to serve as designated decision makers, then the patient needs to appoint a decision maker. Hoffman (1994, p. 239) states, "Surrogate decision makers do not base judgments on their own values, but rather, must endeavor to make choices based upon the patient's previously expressed directives or knowledge of her (his) unique preferences and values." However, Stephens and Grady (1992) state that the durable power of attorney cannot overturn the clear previous expression of a terminally ill person not to be resuscitated.

Patients' rights include both the consent to medical care and the right to withdraw such consent. This, then, becomes the right to die. This right is frequently argued against by physicians and other health personnel. Regelson (1983, p. 95) says it should not be easy for us to let the sick die; we must hold to our image as advocates for life. The rights of terminally ill patients are many, but most important is the right to know the different medical procedures available and the physician's preference for treatment. The patient has the right to autonomy over his or her own body. The patient has a right to express his or her wishes about the use of heroic measures for continuing life and to expect those wishes to be respected. Abrams (1983, p. 94) says although durable health directives are helpful, they are not enough. Each decision has to be explored anew with each patient. Abrams states that right-to-die legislation implies the plug can be pulled without legal vulnerability. She further notes that the quality of life in the last months is meaningful for the sick person and that we must start from a base of optimism and be permitted to pull the plug only as a last resort.

RECENT MEDICAL INTERVENTIONS
OF THE LATTER PART
OF THE TWENTIETH CENTURY

The advent of fertility treatments that produce multiple births, transplants of animal organs into humans, cloning of animals and someday possibly humans, and genetic engineering—these types of medical interventions raise ethical issues for social workers, families, physicians, nurses, and other health care workers.

The debate can begin even before conception. Sperm taken soon after death and frozen can be used years later to produce a child. An egg can be fertilized in vitro, and a woman old enough to be a grandmother can bear a child made from such a fertilized egg.

Organ transplants are common—heart, lungs, and kidneys—but the distribution system is in question. The federal government wants organs to go to the sickest patients first, no matter where they live. Some states have passed laws to keep donated organs within the state borders, no matter the urgency of need elsewhere.

The concepts of death with dignity and physician-assisted dying have been very much in the public arena. Partly, this has been encouraged by Dr. Jack Kevorkian and his many interventions at the request of patients in pain and with terminal conditions. This issue has been placed on the ballot in Oregon and passed by a public vote. This issue raises ethical questions about who makes decisions and the possibility of abuse by family or health workers.

A very tough ethical issue is that of mapping the human genome, essentially the genetic blueprint. It is a good thing to use genes to cure specific illnesses, or to counsel families on the meaning of genetics for certain life decisions. Dr. Sidney Korenman, Associate Dean for Ethics and Medical Science Training at the University of California at Los Angeles (UCLA) said, "It's one thing to insert a gene to prevent fatal illness. It's another thing to select genetic makeups" (Greenberg, 1999, p. 2). Yet we know that the understanding of genes is changing the practice of medicine. Sometimes it is difficult to fully understand biological and medical advancements such as genetic engineering. However, it can provide incredible benefits. Thus, social workers must keep abreast of these issues and be clear about how they feel and the need to assist patients and families to make decisions with which they will be comfortable.

REFLECTIONS AND POSSIBILITIES

A social worker in a New York State hospital described his work with dying patients as very draining:

> It is hard for me because of personal difficulty in terms of the emotional stuff stirred up for me, and it takes its toll. I also have trouble when these emotions are stirred up in colleagues, physicians, and nurses who are not emotionally oriented to these feelings, such as a physician who will not let me, the social worker, get involved. For me it's a lonely kind of work.

He is the only social worker in this hospital. This worker's comment suggests we all need one another. He feels he has limited resources to do his job, and when it involves a dying patient, he has to struggle with difficult physicians. If a social worker is alone in a hospital or a skilled nursing facility, he or she is severely limited in how much time or effort can be devoted to individual dying patients. If there is only one social worker, the facility is more than likely pushing for high productivity from all health personnel, and the dying patient can often receive the least attention of anyone in the facility. Thus, the isolated worker in such a facility may be able to do little to change the isolation of dying patients. The worker's experience just described highlights the isolation of many terminally ill patients in such a setting.

This social worker runs groups with the nurses who feel overwhelmed. Groups are a natural structure for helping persons who feel isolated, overwhelmed, and helpless when transitioning from working with a dying patient to dealing with the patient's death. This was discussed in Chapters 4 and 5. In this case, it is the staff who need help. The group modality returns control to members who feel helpless and dependent.

Social work directors and supervisors should be role models for new workers, demonstrating a willingness to be involved with helping workers understand the needs of dying patients. As workers become more comfortable in a setting, they should be encouraged to become involved with dying patients. Additionally, supervisors must provide respite to workers whose clients are predominantly dying patients and their families. The worker has to feel comfortable with terminally ill and/or bereaved persons, which comes from experience and from coming to terms with one's own mortality. Social workers need to be able to deal with their own anxieties before they can counsel the dying patient (Harper, 1977, p. 100).

A hospice social worker from a New Jersey hospital reported that her first experience was as a student at Sloan Kettering Memorial Hospital working with the parents of terminally ill children:

> I was twenty-two years old, and I almost couldn't bear it. It was one of the hardest things I ever did, and I couldn't wait to get out of there. It was more than I could handle. Two years ago, while working at Paterson General Hospital, I was a co-leader with a nurse doing group therapy with cancer patients. I liked it, and it felt good. There were many rewards, and I had no difficulty in handling my own emotions. I came to this hospice job four months ago and had some reservations. However, I have found it to be the most rewarding and exhilarating experience I have had in the twelve years I've been a social worker.

One can speculate that a twenty-two-year-old social work student who had to deal with terminally ill children would have identification problems. Hospital pediatric units often include patients nineteen and twenty years old. Nevertheless, whatever happened to this student in her field placement at Sloan Kettering Memorial Hospital, she gained knowledge and skills that stood her in good stead for both hospital and hospice work with terminally ill clients. This worker became comfortable working with people and could then extend her comfort to work with dying patients.

A social worker in a hospice setting, a skilled nursing facility, a small hospital, an oncology department of a large hospital, a pediatric oncology unit of a large hospital, or a visiting nurse agency is often the only social worker employed. Such solitary workers need one another and should meet to process their frustrations, feelings, and experiences, good and bad. A group of four hospice social workers in the Albany, New York, area reported on a monthly peer support group they developed for themselves. Group members said the purpose of their group was to reduce isolation, discuss difficult cases, raise ethical issues, engage in problem solving, discuss how they felt about time running out for patients, and clarify roles of other team members. Each of the social workers represented the only worker in the hospice in that area (Blanchard et al., 1984).

This is one way social workers use one another to help themselves and the patients and families with whom they work. The social workers who are employed in hospices are frequently experienced workers who understand the benefits of peer support groups. There is a need for social workers in skilled nursing facilities to meet with oncology workers, for workers in small hospitals to meet with hospice workers, and for social workers in visiting nurse agencies to meet with hospital workers. The purpose is to break out of a particular setting and connect to social workers who work with terminally ill patients as part of their caseload as well as to provide support to those workers whose caseload is made up totally of terminally ill clients.

It is also important for social workers to know that one can always encounter a dying client in an area outside the health field. A school social worker must keep in mind that a child's behavior could be related to a seriously ill or dying relative. A child of thirteen died while practicing basketball in San Diego in October 1999. Events such as this are shocking to fellow students and staff. A social worker in a psychiatric hospital ought to keep in mind that clients' behavior, whether it is decompensation or acting out, can be caused by sick or dying relatives. Since loss and separation are major life themes, they need to be explored in particular with clients to search for the possibility of an impending loss or a recent loss. I know of a social work student who was placed at a labor union's personal counseling center and had a client on her caseload with terminal cancer. The client's family lived in another country, and the illness left him very isolated. In the case of a student, it is possible to bring up the case in class and get help from students placed in health settings. They may be able to share what they do and some of the resources available to cancer patients, perhaps helping students to use e-mail to contact relatives. It can be assumed that social workers in all settings may encounter dying clients or family members who have dying relatives. Since they do not always have colleagues in health care settings available who can assist them, it seems crucial for social workers in health care settings to share their knowledge with the overall social work community.

One social worker who served many years on a pediatric oncology ward of a hospital took a six-month leave of absence and returned to her job with renewed vigor and diminished stress. She called it a mental health leave and posed the question of whether a leave for social workers who work daily with terminal illness should be mandatory, or at least encouraged periodically (Lindamood, 1981). Such a question suggests the notion of burnout, and Caverly (1982), who examines how social workers cope with the terminally ill, compares the coping stages to burnout stages. Burnout stages are listed as follows: enthusiasm, stagnation, frustration, and apathy. Coping stages discussed earlier from Harper's (1977) study are listed as: defensive coping, struggle, ambivalence, and actualized coping. The point is that social workers who work with terminally ill clients do not experience burnout but develop coping mechanisms to help them provide service. Caverly only gathered information from hospital workers, and she suggests her efforts should be expanded to skilled nursing facilities and hospice settings.

The answer to the foregoing questions could come as a result of further examination of settings that are concerned about how their staff interact with dying patients. Tests could be administered to social workers when they begin their employment or placement and, using the same instruments, readministered at regular intervals over a period of time. The results would provide further data with which to make conclusions concerning the association between the services provided by social workers, the setting, and the response of patients and families.

Research needs to be carried out that will help establish guidelines for all professionals who provide services to dying patients and their families. But we must not forget the art of practice. Art is very much a part of medical, nursing, and social work practice.

Some of the areas that come under the rubric of art might be caring, self-awareness, honesty, and compassion. These are qualities that cannot be easily measured and yet are essential when working with dying patients.

Robinson and Billings (1985, p. 214) comment that the acquisition of the personal quality of compassion is not easily taught. They say it depends upon role modeling, "but the role modeling of humanism is doomed to failure unless it is practiced daily by a majority of the faculty." Their plea is directed at physicians and the way they treat their sick and dying patients. Nevertheless, the idea of humanistic and holistic medical practice comes out of a human need that has gone unmet until 1985, when hospice began to expand across the country. The hospice concept and the flood of material related to death and dying is a response to that unmet need. Social workers have been aware of these unmet needs for many years. Social workers and other health professionals have available today tools and knowledge to work more effectively with terminally ill patients and families. Unfortunately, a recent study indicates that terminally ill cancer patients rarely get straight answers from their physicians. Researchers found that doctors are likely to be overly optimistic about their patients' outlooks or simply refuse to comment. Only about one-third are willing to give patients their best guess (Haney, 2000).

The whole question of death and dying underwent abrupt changes in the last decade of the twentieth century, with killings such as the 1995 bombing in Oklahoma City; the 1999 shootings at Columbine High School in Littleton, Colorado; the 1999 shootings in Granada Hills, California of small children because they were Jewish, and of a postal worker because he was not white; the 1998 killing of a nine-year-old boy in Oceanside, California, by someone without any reason whatsoever—the list could go on, but the point about randomness is clear. There is no way to prepare for such mayhem or to protect oneself from such horrors. Social workers have joined forces with other helping professionals to set up teams to go to areas after such disasters to lend assistance to the survivors.

We struggle constantly to construct meaningfulness out of our daily happenings. According to phenomenological theory, human beings cannot exist in a world in which there is no meaning. How do the people of Turkey ascribe meaning to the 1999 earthquake that killed thousands of people, destroying entire families and leaving thousands homeless? Where are the people who constructed the housing which collapsed in the earthquake? It is important to understand the idea that in response to the damaging experiences of reality, human beings struggle to reorder their reality to accommodate something that previously did not fit into their understanding of the world. Braun and Berg (1994) say that all social reality is precious. The constructed reality is in constant threat of collapse. There is always the possibility of a crisis, which can be an event that cannot be explained.

The randomness of much violent death, as discussed in this book, often stresses the need to construct a meaningful event of such experiences. The question "Why?" must be answered in order to construct meaningfulness. This is the largest problem presented to social workers as we begin a new century.

CONCLUSION

It is hoped that social workers who absorb this material will feel comfortable and ready to help dying patients and families and survivors who have lost loved ones to trauma. Although death is the final transition, the process one goes through to arrive there can be one of opportunity rather than dread. Social workers in all settings should be able to use the information provided in this book to assist clients who are coping with life-threatening illnesses and also to help survivors of a loved one's sudden death. Death is a part of life, and helping people to cope with living and teaching people to live fully while dying are important functions of the social work professional.

Bibliography

Abrams, R.D. (1983). Patient rights and responsibilities in irreversible disease. In A.H. Kutscher et al. (Eds.), *Hospice U.S.A.* New York: Columbia University Press.

American Psychiatric Association (1980). *Diagnostic and statistical manual of mental disorders,* Third edition. Washington, DC: American Psychiatric Association.

Anger, I. (1981). Coping with widowhood: A group approach. *Social Work with Groups, Proceedings 1979 Symposium.* Louisville, Kentucky: Committee for the Advancement of Groups.

Annas, G.J. (1985). When procedures limit rights: From Quinlan to Conroy. *The Hastings Center Report, 15*(April), 24-26.

Barry, M.J. (1973). The prolonged grief reaction. *Mayo Clinic Proceedings, 48,* 329-335.

Bartlett, H. (1961). *Social work practice in the health field.* Washington, DC: National Association of Social Workers.

Barton, D. (Ed.) (1977). *Dying and death.* Baltimore: Williams and Wilkins.

Bender, S.J. (1987). The clinical challenge of hospital-based social work practice. *Social Work in Health Care, 13*(2), 25-34.

Benoliel, J.Q. (1971). Assessments of loss and grief. *Journal of Thanatology, 1,* 182-195.

Bernard, J.S. and Schneider, M. (1996). *The true work of dying.* New York: Avon Books.

Bernstein, J.R. (1997). *When the bough breaks: Forever after the death of a son or daughter.* Kansas City, MO: Andrews and McMeel.

Berry, P.E. and Ward, S.E. (1995). Barriers to pain management in hospice: A study of family caregivers. *The Hospice Journal, 10*(4), pp. 19-35.

Bertman, S.L. (1980). Lingering terminal illness and the family: Insights from literature. *Family Process, 19,* 341-348.

Blacher, R.S. (1987). The pain of the physician. *Loss, Grief and Care, 1,* 41-44.

Blanchard, C. et al. (1984). *Professional isolation in oncology and hospice care: Does social work support group help?* Paper presented at NASW Health Conference, Washington, DC, June 11.

Bowlby, J. (1960). Separation anxiety. *International Journal of Psychoanalysis, 41,* parts 2 and 3, 89-113.

Bowlby, J. (1960-1961). Separation anxiety: A critical review of the literature. *Journal of Child Psychology and Psychiatry, 1,* 251-269.

Bowlby, J. (1961). Process of mourning. *International Journal of Psychoanalysis, 42,* parts 3 and 4.

Braun, M.J. and Berg, D.A. (1994). Meaning reconstruction in the experience of parental bereavement. *Death Studies, 18*(2), 105-129.

Brill, N.I. (1976). *Teamwork: Working together in the human services.* New York: J.B. Lippincott-Harper and Row Publishers.

Buckingham, S.L. and Van Gorp, W.G. (1988). Essential knowledge about AIDS dementia. *Social Work, 33.*

Cabot, R.C. (1915). *Social service and the art of healing.* New York: Moffat, Yard and Co.

Cabot, R.C. (1919). *Social work: Essays on the meeting ground of doctor and social worker.* Boston: Houghton-Mifflin Co.

Cairl, R.E. and Kosberg, J.I. (1993). The interface of burden and level of task performance in caregivers of Alzheimer's disease patients: An examination of clinical profiles. *Journal of Gerontological Social Work, 196*(2/3), 133-151.

Calkins, K. (1971). Shouldering a burden. In R.A. Kalish (Ed.), *Caring relationships: The dying and the bereaved.* New York: Baywood Publishing Co.

Caplan, G. (1974). *Support systems and community mental health: Lectures on concept development.* New York: Behavioral Publications.

Cassileth, B.R. and Stinnett, J. (1982). Psychological problems and communication in terminal care. In B.R. Cassileth and P.A. Cassileth (Eds.), *Clinical care of the terminal cancer patient.* Philadelphia: Lea and Febiger.

Caverly, M. (1982). *Coping mechanisms of social work practitioners dealing with the terminally ill.* Paper presented at NASW Clinical Conference, Washington, DC, November 19.

Cho, C. and Cassidy, D.F. (1994). Parallel processes for workers and their clients in chronic bereavement resulting from HIV. *Death Studies, 18*(3), 273-292.

Clayton, P., Desmarais, L., and Winokur, G. (1968). A study of normal bereavement. *American Journal of Psychiatry, 125,* 168-178.

Clayton, P., Desmarais, L., and Winokur, G. (1974). Mourning and depression: Their similarities and differences. *Canadian Psychiatric Association Journal, 19,* 309-312.

Cohen, K.P. (1979). *Hospice.* Germantown, MD: Aspen Systems Corp.

Corr, C.A. and Corr, D.M. (1983). *Hospice care: Principles and practice.* New York: Springer Publishing Co.

Covill, F.J. (1968). Bereavement—A public health challenge. *Canadian Journal of Public Health, 59,* 169-170.

Daeffler, R.J. (1985). A framework for hospice nursing. *The Hospice Journal, 1*(2), 91-111.

DiGiulio, R. and Krantz, R. (1995). *Straight talk about death and dying.* New York: Facts on File.

Doka, K.J. (Ed.) (1996). *Living with grief after sudden loss.* Washington, DC: Hospice Foundation of America.

Doyle, D.G., Hanks, G.W.C., and MacDonald, N. (1993). *Oxford textbook of palliative medicine.* Oxford, U.K.: Oxford University Press.

Drew, F.L. (1986-1987). Suffering and autonomy. *Loss, Grief and Care, 1.*

Dyer, A.R. (1986). Patients, not costs, come first. *Hastings Center Report, 16,* 5-7.

Edmonds, S. and Hooker, K. (1994). Perceived changes in life meaning following bereavement. *Death Studies, 25*(4), 307-308.

Eliot, T.D. (1930a). Bereavement as a problem for family research and technique. *The Family, 11,* 114-115.

Eliot, T.D. (1930b). Family bereavement: A new field for research. *American Sociological Society, 24,* 265-266.

Eliot, T.D. (1932). The bereaved family. *The Annals of the American Academy of Political and Social Sciences, 160,* 184-190.

Eliot, T.D. (1933). A step toward the social psychology of bereavement. *Journal of Abnormal and Social Psychology, 27,* 380-390.

Engel, G.L. (1961). Is grief a disease? *Psychosomatic Disease, 23,* 18-22.

Fackelmann, K. (1999). Survey supports pain-free living for dying patients. *USA Today,* March 18.

Feifel, H. (Ed.) (1977). *New meanings of death.* New York: McGraw-Hill.

Feiger, S.M. and Schmitt, M.H. (1979). Collegiality in interdisciplinary health teams: Its measurement and its effects. *Social Science and Medicine, 13A,* 217-229.

Flannery, R.B. (1997). *Violence in America.* New York: The Continuum Publishing Co.

Flexner, J.M. (1977). Dying, death and the front line physician. In D. Barton (Ed.), *Dying and death: A clinical guide for caregivers* (pp. 170-182). Baltimore: Williams and Wilkins.

Foster, Z. (1979). Standards of hospice care: Assumptions and principles. *Health and Social Work, 4,* 117-128.

Friel, P.B. (1985). Death and dying. In P. Rabin and D. Rabin (Eds.), *To provide safe passage.* New York: Philosophical Library.

Gartner, A. and Reissman, F. (1984). *The self-help revolution.* New York: Human Sciences Press.

Germain, C. (1980). Social work identity competence and autonomy. *Social Work in Health Care, 6*(1), 1-10.

Germain, C.B. (1984). *Social work practice in health care.* New York: The Free Press.

Ginzburg, L.H. (1977). The social worker's role. In E.R. Pritchard et al. (Eds.), *Social work with the dying patient and the family.* New York: Columbia University Press.

Glaser, B. and Strauss, A. (1966). *Awareness of dying.* New York: Aldine.

Glaser, B. and Strauss, A. (1968). *Time for dying.* New York: Aldine.

Goldberg, R. and Tull, R.M. (1983). *The psychosocial dimensions of cancer.* New York: The Free Press.

Goldstein, E. (1973). Social casework and the dying patient. *Social Casework, 54*(10), 601-608.

Goleman, D. (1985). Mourning: New studies affirm its benefits. *The New York Times,* February 5, Sec. C, p. 2.

Gonda, T.A. and Ruark, J.E. (1984). *Dying dignified.* Menlo Park, CA: Addison-Wesley Publishing Co.

Gorer, G. (1965). *Death, grief, and mourning.* Garden City, NY: Doubleday and Co.

Graham, J. (1985). Anger as freedom. In D. Rabin and P. Rabin (Eds.), *To provide safe passage.* New York: Philosophical Library.

Gray-Toft, P. and Anderson, J.G. (1983). Hospice care: A better way of caring for the living. In A.H. Kutscher et al. (Eds.), *Hospice U.S.A.* New York: Columbia University Press.

Greenberg, B. (1999). Medical strides of the 20th century produce ethical quandaries. *North County Times,* April 15, Sec. E, pp. 1-2.

Hamric, A.B. (1977). Deterrents to therapeutic care of the dying person—a nurse's perspective. In D. Barton (Ed.), *Death and dying* (pp. 183-199). Baltimore: Williams and Wilkins.

Haney, D.Q. (2000). "Terminally ill patients often get 'overly optimistic' prognosis." *North County Times,* May 21, 2000, p. A-13.

Harper, B.C. (1977). *Death: The coping mechanism of the health professional.* Greenville, SC: Southeastern University Press.

Harris, M. (1995). *The loss that is forever.* New York: Dutton.

Harris, P.B. (1993). The misunderstood caregiver: A qualified study of the male caregiver of Alzheimer's disease. *The Gerontologist, 33*(4), 551-556.

Hauser, M.J. and Feinberg, D.R. (1976). An operational approach to the delayed grief and mourning process. *Journal of Psychiatric Nursing and Mental Health Services, 14,* 29-35.

Henderson, E. (1972). The approach to the patient with an incurable disease. In B. Schoenberg, A.C. Carr, D. Peretz, and A.H. Katsch (Eds.), *Psychosocial aspects of terminal care* (pp. 57-61). New York: Columbia University Press.

Hersh, S.P. (1996). After heart attack and stroke. In K.J. Doka (Ed.), *Living with grief after sudden loss.* Washington, DC: Hospice Foundation of America.

Hill, R. (1967). Generic features of families under stress. In H.J. Parad (Ed.), *Crisis intervention.* New York: Columbia University Press.

Hoagland, A.C. (1984). *Bereavement and personal construct conceptualization.* Washington, DC: Hemisphere Publishing Co.

Hodge, J.R. (1971). Help your patients to mourn better. *Medical Times, 99,* 53-64.

Hoffman, M.K. (1994). Advance directives: A social work perspective on the myth versus the reality. *Death Studies, 18*(3), 229-241.

Johnston, W.I. (1995). *HIV negative: How the uninfected are affected by AIDS.* New York: Insight Books Plenum Press.

Kalish, R.A. (1971). *Caring relationships: The dying and the bereaved.* New York: Baywood Publishing Co.

Kamerman, J.B. (1988). *Death in the midst of life.* Englewood Cliffs, NJ: Prentice-Hall.

Kane, R.A. (1982). Terms: Thoughts from the bleachers. *Health and Social Work, 7,* 2-4.

Kastenbaum, R. (1979). Healthy dying: A paradoxical quest continues. *Journal of Social Issues, 35*(1), 185-206.

Kastenbaum, R. and Aisenberg, R. (1976). *The psychology of death.* New York: Springer Publishing Co.

Katz, B.P., Zdeb, M.S., and Therriault, G.D. (1979). Where people die. *Public Health Reports, 94,* 522-527.

Katzman, R., Hill, R., and Esh, Y. (1994). The malignancy of dementia predictors of mortality in clinically diagnosed dementia in a population survey of Shanghai, China. *Archives of Neurology, 151,* 1220-1225.

Kleinman, D. (1985). Hospital care of the dying: Each day painful choices. *The New York Times,* January 14, Sec. B, p. 4.

Koff, T.H. (1980). *Hospice: A caring community.* Cambridge, MA: Winthrop Publishers.

Krant, M.J. (1972). The organized care of the dying patient. *Hospital Practice, 7,* 101-108.

Krant, M.J. (1973). Grief and bereavement: An unmet medical need. *Delaware Medical Journal, 45,* 282-290.

Kübler-Ross, E. (1969). *On death and dying.* New York: Macmillan, Inc.

Kustoborder, J.J. (1980). Multidisciplinary committee identifies high risk patients, coordinates care. *Hospital Progress, 61,* 63-65, 70.

Lack, S.A. and Buckingham, R.W. (1978). *The first American hospice.* New Haven, CT: Hospice, Inc.

Landes, A., Siegel, M.A., and Foster, C.D. (1994). *Death and dying—Who decides* (pp. 79-100). Wylie, TX: Information Plus.

Lee, S. (1980). Interdisciplinary teaming in primary care: A process of evolution and resolution. *Social Work in Health Care, 5,* 237-244.

Levine, A.S. (1985). The doctor-patient relationship in oncology: Implications for practice, research, and policy planning. In S.C. Gross and S. Garb (Eds.), *Cancer treatment and research in humanistic perspective.* New York: Springer Publishing Co.

Levinson, P. (1975). Obstacles in the treatment of dying patients. *American Journal of Psychiatry, 132,* 28-32.

Lifton, R.J. (1979). *The broken connection.* New York: Simon and Schuster.

Likert, R. (1967). *The human organization.* New York: McGraw-Hill.

Lindamood, M.M. (1981). Leave means never having to say I quit. *Social Work in Health Care, 7*(2), 101-103.

Lindeman, E. (1944). Symptomatology and management of acute grief. *American Journal of Psychiatry, 101,* 141-148.

Lister, L. (1982). Role training for interdisciplinary health teams. *Health and Social Work, 7*(1), 19-25.

Liu, Y. (1983). Death and dying fear patterns in children's hospital social workers. *La Travailler—The Social Worker, 51,* 7-10.

Lohmann, R.A. (1979). Dying and the social responsibility of institutions. *Social Casework, 58,* 538-545.

Lord, J.H. (1996). America's number one killer: Vehicular crashes. In K.J. Doka (Ed.), *Living with grief after sudden loss* (pp. 25-39). Washington, DC: Hospice Foundation of America.

Lowe, J.I. and Herranen, M. (1981). Understanding teamwork: Another look at the concepts. *Social Work in Health Care, 7.*

McCollum, A.T. and Schwartz, H.S. (1972). Social work and the mourning patient. *Social Work, 17,* 25-36.

McDonnell, A. (1986). *Quality hospice care.* Owings Mills, MD: National Health Publishing.

McIntosh, J.L. (1993). Control group studies of suicide survivors: A review and critique. *Suicide and Life Threatening Behavior, 23*(2).

Mor, V. (1987). *Hospice care systems.* New York: Springer Publishing Co.

Mor, V. and Hiris, J. (1983). Determinants of site of death among cancer patients. *Journal of Health and Social Behavior, 24*(2), 375-385.

Morgan, N. (1999). Now doctors visit hospice to learn care for the dying. *San Diego Union Tribune,* March 9, p. A3.

Munley, A. (1983). *The hospice alternative.* New York: Basic Books.

NASW News (May, 1988).

New, P.K. (1965). Another approach to professionalism. *American Journal of Nursing, 65,* 124-126.

New, P.K. (1968). An analysis of the concept of teamwork. *Community Mental Health Journal, 4,* 326-337.

Olson, K.W. (1988, May). Hospice care as presented by the Shanti Project of San Francisco. San Jose State University, School of Social Work, unpublished paper.

Orcutt, B.A. (1977). Stress in family interaction when a member is dying: A special case for family interviews. In E. Pritchard et al. (Eds.), *Social work with the dying patient and family.* New York: Columbia University Press.

Paridis, L.F. (1985). *Hospice handbook: A guide for managers and planners.* Rockville, MD: Aspen Publications.

Parkes, C.M. (1970). Seeking and finding a lost object. *Social Science and Medicine, 4,* 187-201.

Parkes, C.M. (1971). Psychosocial transitions: A field of study. *Social Science and Medicine, 5,* 101-115.

Parkes, C.M. (1972). Health after bereavement—A controlled study of young Boston widows and widowers. *Psychosomatic Medicine, 34,* 449-461.

Parkes, C.M. (1975). Determinants of outcome following bereavement. *Omega, 6,* 303-323.

Parkes, C.M. and Weiss, R.S. (1983). *Recovery from bereavement.* New York: Basic Books.

Parliament of Victoria, Social Development Committee (1987, April). *Inquiring into options for dying with dignity* (Second final report). Melbourne, Victoria, Australia.

Parry, J.K. (1983). *Social workers and the terminally ill: Social workers' feelings about clients, job satisfaction, and organizational settings.* Dissertation, Yeshiva University, New York City.

Parry, J.K. (1990). *Social work practice with the terminally ill: The transcultural perspective.* Springfield, IL: Charles C Thomas Publishing.

Parry, J.K. (1995). *A cross-cultural look at death, dying, and religion.* Chicago, IL: Nelson-Hall Publishers.

Parry, J.K. and Kahn, N. (1976). Group work with emphysema patients. *Social Work in Health Care, 2*(1), 55-64.

Pattison, E.M. (1977). *The experience of dying.* Englewood Cliffs, NJ: Prentice-Hall.

Peeples, E.H. and Francis, G.M. (1968). Social-psychological obstacles to effective health team practice. *Nursing Forum, 7,* 28-37.

Pendarvis, J.F. and Grinnel, R.M. (1980). The use of a rehabilitation team for stroke patients. *Social Work in Health Care, 6,* 2.

Pilsecker, C. (1975). Help for the dying. *Social Work, 20*(3), 190-199.

Powers, L.E. and Wampold, B.E. (1994). Cognitive-behavioral factors in adjustment to adult bereavement. *Death Studies, 18*(1), 1-24.

Proffitt, L. (1985). Management of the hospice home care program. In L.F. Paradis (Ed.), *Hospice handbook* (pp. 173-190). Rockville, MD: Aspen Publications.

Rabin, D. and Rabin, P.L. (1985). *To provide safe passage.* New York: Philosophical Library.

Rabin, P.L. and Pate, K.J. (1985). Acute grief. In D. Rabin and P.L. Rabin (Eds.), *To provide safe passage.* New York: Philosophical Library.

Rae-Grant, Q.A.F. and Marcuse, D.J. (1968). The hazards of teamwork. *American Journal of Orthopsychiatry, 38,* 4-8.

Rapoport, R. (1966). Normal crises, family structure, and mental health. In H.J. Parad (Ed.), *Crisis intervention.* New York: Columbia University Press.

Raven, R.W. (1985). The development and practice of oncology. In S.C. Gross and S. Garb (Eds.), *Cancer treatment and research in humanistic perspective.* New York: Springer Publishing Co.

Reamer, F.G. (1985). Facing up to the challenge of DRGs. *Health and Social Work, 10*(2), 85-94.

Redmond, L.M. (1996). Sudden violent death. In K.J. Doka (Ed.), *Living with grief after sudden loss* (pp. 53-71). Washington, DC: Hospice Foundation of America.

Rees, D.W. and Lutkins, S.G. (1967). Mortality and bereavement. *British Medical Journal, 4,* 13-16.

Regelson, W. (1983). Death with dignity. In A.H. Kutscher, S.C. Klagsbrun, R.J. Torpie, R. DeBellis, M.S. Hale, and M. Tallmer (Eds.), *Hospice U.S.A.* (pp. 88-95). New York: Columbia University Press.

Richard, E. and Shepard, A.C. (1981). Giving up smoking: A lesson in loss theory. *American Journal of Nursing,* April, 755-757.

Robinson, R.R. and Billings, F.T. (1985). Some reflections on humanism in medicine. In D. Rabin and P.L. Rabin (Eds.), *To provide safe passage.* New York: Philosophical Library.

Rodman, H. and Kolodny, R.L. (1965). Organizational strains in the research-practitioner relationship. In A.W. Gouldner and S.M. Miller (Eds.), *Applied sociology: Opportunities and problems.* New York: The Free Press.

Ross, E. (1993). Preventing burnout among social workers employed in the field of AIDS/HIV. *Social Work in Health Care, 18*(2), 91-108.

Russell, R. (1977). *Freedom to die,* Revised edition. New York: Human Sciences Press.

Ryder, C.F. and Ross, D.H. (1977). Terminal care: Issues and alternatives. *Public Health Reports, 92,* 20-29.

Schnaper, N., Kellner, T.K., and Koeppel, B. (1985). Doctors and cancer patients. In P. Rabin and D. Rabin (Eds.), *To provide safe passage.* New York: Philosophical Library.

Schwartz, A.M. and Karusu, T.B. (1977). Psychotherapy with the dying patient. *American Journal of Psychotherapy, 31*(1), 19-35.

Seplowin, V.M. and Seravilli, E. (1983). The hospice: Its changes through time. In A.H. Kutscher, S.C. Klagsbrun, R.J. Torpie, R. DeBellis, M.S. Hale, and M. Tallmer (Eds.), *Hospice U.S.A.* (pp. 3-8). New York: Columbia University Press.

Shrader, D. (1986). On dying more than one death. *Hastings Center Report, 16,* 12-17.

Silverman, P.R. and Worden, J.W. (1992). Children's understanding of funeral ritual. *Omega, 25*(4), 319-331.

Sinacore, J.M. (1981). Avoiding the humanistic aspect of death, an outcome from the implicit elements of health professors education. *Death Education, 5,* 121-133.

Stephens, R.L. and Grady, R. (1992). Case analyses of terminally ill cancer patients who refused to sign a Living Will. *Omega, 25*(4), 283-289.

Stillion, J.M. (1996). Survivors of suicide. In K.J. Doka (Ed.), *Living with grief after sudden loss* (pp. 41-51). Washington, DC: Hospice Foundation of America.

Stoddard, S. (1978). *The hospice movement.* New York: First Vantage Books.

Strauss, A.L. and Glaser, B.G. (1970). Patterns of dying. In O.G. Brim Jr. et al. (Eds.), *The dying patient.* New York: Russell Sage.

Strauss, A., Glaser, B., and Quint, J. (1964). The non-accountability of terminal care. *Hospitals, 38.*

Stubblefield, K.S. (1977). A preventive program for bereaved families. *Social Work in Health Care, 2*(4), 379-389.

Twycross, R.G. (1975). The use of narcotic analgesics in terminal illness. *Journal of Medical Ethics, 1,* 10-17.

Uroda, S.F. (1977). Counseling the bereaved. *Counseling and Values, 21,* 185-191.

U.S. program offers dying alternatives to hospital care. *The New York Times,* November 6, 1983, Sec. 1, p. 32.

Vachon, M.L.S. (1976). Grief and bereavement following the death of a spouse. *Canadian Psychiatric Association Journal, 21,* 35-44.

Veatch, R. (1972). Brain death: Welcome definition or dangerous adjustment? *Hastings Center Report, 2*(November), 10-13.

Vess, J.D., Moreland, J.R., and Schwebel, A.I. (1985). An empirical assessment of the effects of cancer on family role functioning. *Journal of Psychosocial Oncology, 3,* 1-14.

Viney, L.L. (1984). Concerns about death among severely ill people. In F.R. Eptin and R.A. Neimeyer (Eds.), *Personal meanings of death* (pp. 143-157). New York: Hemisphere Publishing Corp.

Wahl, C.W. (1970). The differential diagnosis of normal and neurotic grief following bereavement. *Psychosomatics, 11,* 104-106.

Weiner, M.F. (1999). Alzheimer's disease update. *Consultant,* March, 675-685.

Weisman, A.D. (1972). *On dying and denying.* New York: Behavioral Publications.

White, R.B. and Gathman, L.T. (1973). The syndrome of ordinary grief. *American Family Physician, 8,* 97-104.

Whitt, J.K. et al. (1981-1982). Pediatric liaison psychiatry: A forum for separation and loss. *International Journal of Psychiatry in Medicine, 11,* 59-68.

Wiener, L.S. and Siegel, L. (1990). Social workers comfort in providing services to AIDS patients. *Social Work, 35*(1), 18-25.

Williams, R.B. et al. (1970). The use of a therapeutic milieu on a continuing care unit in a general hospital. *Annals of Internal Medicine, 73,* 957-962.

Wilson, D.C., Ajemian, I., and Mount, B.M. (1978). Montreal (1975), The Royal Victoria Hospital palliative care service. In G.W. Davidson (Ed.), *The hospice.* Washington, DC: Hemisphere Publishing Corp.

Wollert, R., Knight, B., and Levy, L.H. (1984). Make today count. In A. Gartner and F. Riessman (Eds.), *The self-help revolution.* New York: Human Sciences Press.

Yolom, I.D. and Vinogrador, S. (1988). Bereavement groups: Techniques and themes. *International Journal of Psychotherapy, 38*(4), 419-445.

Zaner, R.M. (1985). A philosopher reflects: A play against night's advance. In D. Rabin and P.L. Rabin (Eds.), *To provide safe passage.* New York: Philosophical Library.

Zimmerman, J.M. (1981). *Hospice: Complete care for the terminally ill.* Baltimore: Urban and Schwarzenberg.

Index

HAWORTH Social Work Practice in Action
Carlton E. Munson, PhD, Senior Editor

SOCIAL WORK THEORY AND PRACTICE WITH THE TERMINALLY ILL by Joan K. Parry (2001). "Whether one wishes to focus on theory or practice, I recommend this excellent, caring book to anyone who wants to meet the challenges of working with the terminally ill and their survivors." *Jean A. Gill, PhD, LCSW, Adjunct Faculty, San Diego State University*

WOMEN SURVIVORS, PSYCHOLOGICAL TRAUMA, AND THE POLITICS OF RESISTANCE by Norma Jean Profitt. (2000). "A compelling argument on the importance of political and collective action as a means of resisting oppression." *Gloria Geller, PhD, Faculty of Social Work, University of Regina, Saskatchewan, Canada*

THE MENTAL HEALTH DIAGNOSTIC DESK REFERENCE: VISUAL GUIDES AND MORE FOR LEARNING TO USE THE DIAGNOSTIC AND STATISTICAL MANUAL (DSM-IV) by Carlton E. Munson. (2000). "A carefully organized and user-friendly book for the beginning student and less-experienced practitioner of social work, clinical psychology, or psychiatric nursing . . . . It will be a valuable addition to the literature on clinical assessment of mental disorders." *Jerrold R. Brandell, PhD, BCD, Professor, School of Social Work, Wayne State University, Detroit, Michigan and Founding Editor,* Psychoanalytic Social Work

HUMAN SERVICES AND THE AFROCENTRIC PARADIGM by Jerome H. Schiele. (2000). "Represents a milestone in applying the Afrocentric paradigm to human services generally, and social work specifically. . . . A highly valuable resource." *Bogart R. Leashore, PhD, Dean and Professor, Hunter College School of Social Work, New York, New York*

SOCIAL WORK: SEEKING RELEVANCY IN THE TWENTY-FIRST CENTURY by Roland Meinert, John T. Pardeck and Larry Kreuger. (2000). "Highly recommended. A thought-provoking work that asks the difficult questions and challenges the status quo. A great book for graduate students as well as experienced social workers and educators." *Francis K. O. Yuen, DSW, ACSE, Associate Professor, Division of Social Work, California State University, Sacramento*

SOCIAL WORK PRACTICE IN HOME HEALTH CARE by Ruth Ann Goode. (2000). "Dr. Goode presents both a lucid scenario and a formulated protocol to bring health care services into the home setting. . . . This is a must have volume that will be a reference to be consulted many times." *Marcia B. Steinhauer, PhD, Coordinator and Associate Professor, Human Services Administration Program, Rider University, Lawrence-ville, New Jersey*

FORENSIC SOCIAL WORK: LEGAL ASPECTS OF PROFESSIONAL PRAC-TICE, SECOND EDITION by Robert L. Barker and Douglas M. Branson. (2000). "The authors combine their expertise to create this informative guide to address legal practice issues facing social workers." *Newsletter of the National Organization of Foren-sic Social Work*

SOCIAL WORK IN THE HEALTH FIELD: A CARE PERSPECTIVE by Lois A. Fort Cowles. (1999). "Makes an important contribution to the field by locating the practice of social work in health care within an organizational and social context." *Goldie Kadushin, PhD, Associate Professor, School of Social Welfare, University of Wisconsin, Milwaukee*

SMART BUT STUCK: WHAT EVERY THERAPIST NEEDS TO KNOW ABOUT LEARNING DISABILITIES AND IMPRISONED INTELLIGENCE by Myrna Orenstein. (1999). "A trailblazing effort that creates an entirely novel way of talking and thinking about learning disabilities. There is simply nothing like it in the field." *Fred M. Levin, MD, Training Supervising Analyst, Chicago Institute for Psychoanalysis; Assistant Professor of Clinical Psychiatry, Northwestern University, School of Medicine, Chicago, IL*

CLINICAL WORK AND SOCIAL ACTION: AN INTEGRATIVE APPROACH by Jerome Sachs and Fred Newdom. (1999). "Just in time for the new millennium come Sachs and Newdom with a wholly fresh look at social work. . . . A much-needed uniting of social work values, theories, and practice for action." *Josephine Nieves, MSW, PhD, Executive Director, National Association of Social Workers*

SOCIAL WORK PRACTICE IN THE MILITARY by James G. Daley. (1999). "A significant and worthwhile book with provocative and stimulating ideas. It deserves to be read by a wide audience in social work education and practice as well as by decision makers in the military." *H. Wayne Johnson, MSW, Professor, University of Iowa, School of Social Work, Iowa City, Iowa*

GROUP WORK: SKILLS AND STRATEGIES FOR EFFECTIVE INTERVENTIONS, SECOND EDITION by Sondra Brandler and Camille P. Roman. (1999). "A clear, basic description of what group work requires, including what skills and techniques group workers need to be effective." *Hospital and Community Psychiatry* (from the first edition)

TEENAGE RUNAWAYS: BROKEN HEARTS AND "BAD ATTITUDES" by Laurie Schaffner (1999). "Skillfully combines the authentic voice of the juvenile runaway with the principles of social science research." *Barbara Owen, PhD, Professor, Department of Criminology, California State University, Fresno*

CELEBRATING DIVERSITY: COEXISTING IN A MULTICULTURAL SOCIETY by Benyamin Chetkow-Yanoov. (1999). "Makes a valuable contribution to peace theory and practice." *Ian Harris, EdD, Executive Secretary, Peace Education Committee, International Peace Research Association*

SOCIAL WELFARE POLICY ANALYSIS AND CHOICES by Hobart A. Burch. (1999). "Will become the landmark text in its field for many decades to come." *Sheldon Rahan, DSW, Founding Dean and Emeritus Professor of Social Policy and Social Administration. Faculty of Social Work, Wilfrid Laurier University, Canada*

SOCIAL WORK PRACTICE: A SYSTEMS APPROACH, SECOND EDITION by Benyamin Chetkow-Yannov. (1999). "Highly recommended as a primary text for any and all introductory social work courses." *Ram A. Cnaan, PhD, Associate Professor, School of Social Work, University of Pennsylvania*

CRITICAL SOCIAL WELFARE ISSUES: TOOLS FOR SOCIAL WORK AND HEALTH CARE PROFESSIONALS edited by Arthur J. Katz, Abraham Lurie, and Carlos M. Vidal. (1997). "Offers hopeful agendas for change, while navigating the societal challenges facing those in the human services today." *Book News Inc.*

SOCIAL WORK IN HEALTH SETTINGS: PRACTICE IN CONTEXT, SECOND EDITION edited by Toba Schwaber Kerson. (1997). "A first-class document . . . It will be found among the steadier and lasting works on the social work aspects of American health care." *Hans S. Falck, PhD, Professor Emeritus and Former Chair, Health Specialization in Social Work, Virginia Commonwealth University*

PRINCIPLES OF SOCIAL WORK PRACTICE: A GENERIC PRACTICE APPROACH by Molly R. Hancock. (1997). "Hancock's discussions advocate reflection and self-awareness to create a climate for client change." *Journal of Social Work Education*

NOBODY'S CHILDREN: ORPHANS OF THE HIV EPIDEMIC by Steven F. Dansky. (1997). "Professional sound, moving, and useful for both professionals and interested readers alike." *Ellen G. Friedman, ACSW, Associate Director of Support Services, Beth Israel Medical Center, Methadone Maintenance Treatment Program*

SOCIAL WORK APPROACHES TO CONFLICT RESOLUTION: MAKING FIGHTING OBSOLETE by Benyamin Chetkow-Yanoov. (1996). "Presents an examination of the nature and cause of conflict and suggests techniques for coping with conflict." *Journal of Criminal Justice*

FEMINIST THEORIES AND SOCIAL WORK: APPROACHES AND APPLICATIONS by Christine Flynn Salunier. (1996). " An essential reference to be read repeatedly by all educators and practitioners who are eager to learn more about feminist theory and practice: *Nancy R. Hooyman, PhD, Dean and Professor, School of Social Work, University of Washington, Seattle*

THE RELATIONAL SYSTEMS MODEL FOR FAMILY THERAPY: LIVING IN THE FOUR REALITIES by Donald R. Bardill. (1996). "Engages the reader in quiet, thoughtful conversation on the timeless issue of helping families and individuals." *Christian Counseling Resource Review*

SOCIAL WORK INTERVENTION IN AN ECONOMIC CRISIS: THE RIVER COMMUNITIES PROJECT by Martha Baum and Pamela Twiss. (1996). "Sets a standard for universities in terms of the types of meaningful roles they can play in supporting and sustaining communities." *Kenneth J. Jaros, PhD, Director, Public Health Social Work Training Program, University of Pittsburgh*

FUNDAMENTALS OF COGNITIVE-BEHAVIOR THERAPY: FROM BOTH SIDES OF THE DESK by Bill Borcherdt. (1996). "Both beginning and experienced practitioners . . . will find a considerable number of valuable suggestions in Borcherdt's book." *Albert Ellis, PhD, President, Institute for Rational-Emotive Therapy, New York City*

BASIC SOCIAL POLICY AND PLANNING: STRATEGIES AND PRACTICE METHODS by Hobart A. Burch. (1996). "Burch's familiarity with his topic is evident and his book is an easy introduction to the field." *Readings*

THE CROSS-CULTURAL PRACTICE OF CLINICAL CASE MANAGEMENT IN MENTAL HEALTH edited by Peter Manoleas. (1996). "Makes a contribution by bringing together the cross-cultural and clinical case management perspectives in working with those who have serious mental illness." *Disability Studies Quarterly*

FAMILY BEYOND FAMILY: THE SURROGATE PARENT IN SCHOOLS AND OTHER COMMUNITY AGENCIES by Sanford Weinstein. (1995). "Highly recommended to anyone concerned about the welfare of our children and the break-down of the American family." *Jerold S. Greenberg, EdD, Director of Community Service, College of Health & Human Performance, University of Maryland*

PEOPLE WITH HIV AND THOSE WHO HELP THEM: CHALLENGES, INTEGRATION, INTERVENTION by R. Dennis Shelby. (1995). "A useful and compassionate contribution to the HIV psychotherapy literature." *Public Health*

THE BLACK ELDERLY: SATISFACTION AND QUALITY OF LATER LIFE by Marguerite Coke and James A. Twaite. (1995). "Presents a model for predicting life satisfaction in this population." *Abstracts in Social Gerontology*

BUILDING ON WOMEN'S STRENGTHS: A SOCIAL WORK AGENDA FOR THE TWENTY-FIRST CENTURY edited by Liane V. Davis. (1994). "The most lucid and accessible overview of the related epistemological debates int he social work literature." *Journal of the National Association of Social Workers*

NOW DARE EVERYTHING: TALES OF HIV-RELATED PSYCHOTHERAPY by Steven F. Dansky. (1994). "A highly recommended book for anyone working with persons who are HIV positive. . . . Every library should have a copy of this book." *AIDS Book Review Journal*

INTERVENTION RESEARCH: DESIGN AND DEVELOPMENT FOR HUMAN SERVICE edited by Jack Rothman and Edwin J. Thomas. (1994). "Provides a useful framework for the further examination of methodology for each separate step of such research." *Academic Library Book Review*

CLINICAL SOCIAL WORK SUPERVISION, SECOND EDITION by Carlton E. Munson. (1993). "A useful, thorough, and articulate reference for supervisors and for 'supervisees' who are wanting to understand their supervisor or are looking for effective supervision." *Transactional Analysis Journal*

ELEMENTS OF THE HELPING PROCESS: A GUIDE FOR CLINICIANS by Raymond Fox. (1993). "Filled with helpful hints, creative interventions, and practical guidelines." *Journal of Family Psychotherapy*

IF A PARTNER HAS AIDS: GUIDE TO CLINICAL INTERVENTION FOR RELATIONSHIPS IN CRISIS by R. Dennis Shelby. (1993). " A welcome addition to existing publications about couples coping with AIDS, it offers intervention ideas and strategies to clinicians." *Contemporary Psychology*

GERONTOLOGICAL SOCIAL WORK SUPERVISION by Ann Burack-Weiss and Frances Coyle Brennan. (1991). "The creative ideas in this book will aid supervisors working with students and experienced social workers." *Senior News*

SOCIAL WORK THEORY AND PRACTICE WITH THE TERMINALLY ILL by Joan K. Parry. (1989). "Should be read by all professionals engaged in the provision of health services in hospitals, emergency rooms, and hospices." *Hector B. Garcia, PhD, Professor, San Jose State University School of Social Work*

THE CREATIVE PRACTITIONER: THEORY AND METHODS FOR THE HELPING SERVICES by Bernard Gelfand. (1988). "[Should] be widely adopted by those in the helping services. It could lead to significant positive advances by countless individuals." *Sidney J. Parnes, Trustee Chairperson for Strategic Program Development, Creative Education Foundation, Buffalo, NY*

MANAGEMENT AND INFORMATION SYSTEMS IN HUMAN SERVICES: IMPLICATIONS FOR THE DISTRIBUTION OF AUTHORITY AND DECISION MAKING by Richard K. Caputo. (1987). "A contribution to social work scholarship in that it provides conceptual frameworks that can be used in the design of management information systems." *Social Work*

Order Your Own Copy of
This Important Book for Your Personal Library!

SOCIAL WORK THEORY AND PRACTICE
WITH THE TERMINALLY ILL, SECOND EDITION

_____ in hardbound at $49.95 (ISBN: 0-7890-1082-8)

_____ in softbound at $24.95 (ISBN: 0-7890-1083-6)

COST OF BOOKS_____

OUTSIDE USA/CANADA/
MEXICO: ADD 20%_____

POSTAGE & HANDLING_____
(US: $4.00 for first book & $1.50
for each additional book
Outside US: $5.00 for first book
& $2.00 for each additional book)

SUBTOTAL_____

IN CANADA: ADD 7% GST_____

STATE TAX_____
(NY, OH & MN residents, please
add appropriate local sales tax)

FINAL TOTAL_____
(If paying in Canadian funds,
convert using the current
exchange rate. UNESCO
coupons welcome.)

☐ **BILL ME LATER:** ($5 service charge will be added)
(Bill-me option is good on US/Canada/Mexico orders only;
not good to jobbers, wholesalers, or subscription agencies.)

☐ Check here if billing address is different from
shipping address and attach purchase order and
billing address information.

Signature_____

☐ **PAYMENT ENCLOSED: $** _____

☐ **PLEASE CHARGE TO MY CREDIT CARD.**

☐ Visa   ☐ MasterCard   ☐ AmEx   ☐ Discover
☐ Diner's Club   ☐ Eurocard   ☐ JCB

Account # _____

Exp. Date _____

Signature _____

Prices in US dollars and subject to change without notice.

NAME _____

INSTITUTION _____

ADDRESS _____

CITY _____

STATE/ZIP _____

COUNTRY _____ COUNTY (NY residents only) _____

TEL _____ FAX _____

E-MAIL_____

May we use your e-mail address for confirmations and other types of information? ☐ Yes   ☐ No
We appreciate receiving your e-mail address and fax number. Haworth would like to e-mail or fax special
discount offers to you, as a preferred customer. **We will never share, rent, or exchange your e-mail
address or fax number.** We regard such actions as an invasion of your privacy.

Order From Your Local Bookstore or Directly From
The Haworth Press, Inc.
10 Alice Street, Binghamton, New York 13904-1580 • USA
TELEPHONE: 1-800-HAWORTH (1-800-429-6784) / Outside US/Canada: (607) 722-5857
FAX: 1-800-895-0582 / Outside US/Canada: (607) 772-6362
E-mail: getinfo@haworthpressinc.com
PLEASE PHOTOCOPY THIS FORM FOR YOUR PERSONAL USE.
www.HaworthPress.com

BOF00